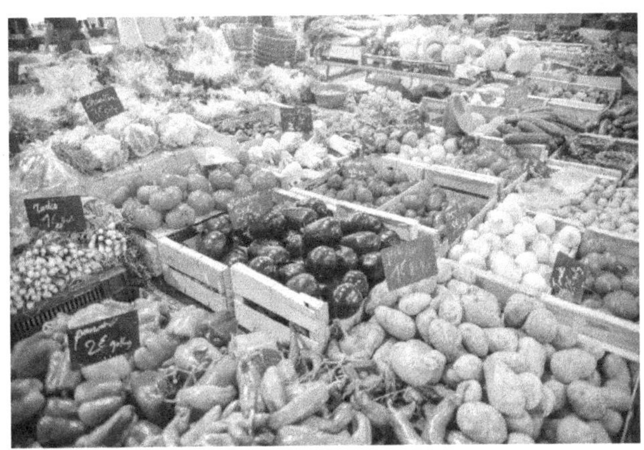

Juicing for Vibrant Health Nourish Your Body and Boost Your Energy with Fresh Juice

Written by
Aimee and Scott Kleppin

ISBN: 9798387538643

Published by Amazon Independently publishing.

In today's fast-paced world, it can be challenging to find the time and energy to take care of ourselves properly. We are constantly bombarded with advertisements for fast food, sugary drinks, and processed snacks that can harm our bodies and minds. However, there is a simple and effective way to nourish your body and boost your energy fresh juice.

In this book, **Juicing for Vibrant Health**, the author shares delicious recipes and practical advice on how to use juicing to reverse diabetes, improve heart health, enhance circulation, cleanse your system, and reverse aging. With its easy-to-follow recipes, this book will guide you step-by-step on how to create healthy and tasty juices that will make you feel rejuvenated and full of vitality.

The author's passion for juicing and commitment to healthy living shines through on every page. This book presents a wealth of information and insights with a warm, enthusiastic tone that reflects a deep understanding of the principles and practices of healthy living. Whether you are new to juicing or a seasoned expert, you will find this book a valuable resource for achieving optimal health and well-being.

I highly recommend **Juicing for Vibrant Health** to anyone who wants to take control of their health, feel energized, and live their best life. Enjoy!

Introduction:

I wrote this book to share my experience with juicing and how it has transformed my health. It all started with the inspiration of fitness legend Jack LaLanne, who swore by the power of juicing. However, like many of us, I neglected my nutrition and lived off unhealthy foods in my 20s, which led to health issues like high blood pressure, high cholesterol, and type 2 diabetes in my 50s.

I tried different diets, but I found it hard to stick to them, and I love my comfort foods. So, I started exploring nutritional options that could help me achieve similar results without feeling like I was constantly depriving myself. That's when I rediscovered the power of juicing.

While some may dismiss juicing as a trendy fad, there is scientific evidence to support its health benefits. For instance, consuming larger quantities of Vitamin C can reduce total cholesterol, and increasing fiber intake through juicing can promote bowel regularity and reduce the risk of colon cancer. Juicing can also be an excellent way to incorporate more leafy greens into your diet, which are rich in vitamins and minerals that can improve overall health. Moreover, juicing has shown great potential in improving heart health issues, which is why the legendary fitness guru Jack LaLanne was a big proponent of juicing.

Juicing has worked wonders for my health, and it doesn't have to feel like a chore. I still eat mostly veggies and avoid bread, but I've added juicing to supercharge my diet. And the best part is that I don't have to avoid the foods I love, as I can still indulge in pizza on Fridays and the occasional dessert. Since I started this journey, my blood pressure has gone down, my cholesterol has greatly improved, and my glucose numbers are in check.

Therefore, I wrote this book to share my personal experience and encourage others to explore the benefits of juicing. As the famous quote by Jack LaLanne goes, *"exercise is king, nutrition is queen, put them together and you've got a kingdom."* And in my kingdom, there's always room for a good juice. In fact, the history of juicing dates to ancient times, and it's fascinating to see how it has evolved over the years to become a popular health trend today.

In the early 1900s, juicing gained popularity in the United States, largely thanks to Dr. Norman Walker, who is known as the "Juice King." He invented the first modern juicing machine, the Norwalk Juicer, and authored multiple books on the health benefits of juicing.

In the 1920s, the popularity of juicing continued to grow, with many Americans turning to fresh juice to improve their health and well-being. This was also the decade when juicing machines became more widely available, making it easier for people to create their own juice at home.

In the 1950s and 1960s, juicing took a backseat to other health trends like diet pills and low-fat diets. However, it continued to be a staple in health food stores and natural living communities.

In the 1970s, juicing became a trendy health practice, as people started experimenting with different fruits and vegetables to create new and delicious juice recipes. Juice bars and health food stores started popping up all over the country, and the natural foods and "hippie" culture of the time further fueled the trend.

In the 1980s and 1990s, juicing experienced a resurgence in popularity, thanks in part to the rise of the health and wellness industry. Celebrities like Gwyneth Paltrow and Oprah Winfrey were vocal proponents of juicing, and juice bars and cafes became popular hangouts for health-conscious individuals.

In the 21st century, juicing has continued to evolve and adapt to changing health trends. Green juices and smoothies have become especially popular, with many people using them to detoxify their bodies and boost their immune systems.

Today, juicing is more popular than ever, with many people turning to fresh juice to enhance their health and energy levels. Social media has further amplified the trend, with a plethora of creative and colorful juice recipes to try.

Welcome to **_Juicing for Vibrant Health_**, a comprehensive guide that will help you harness the power of fresh juice to regenerate your body, mind, and spirit. In today's world, we face many challenges that can deplete our energy and vitality, from unhealthy diets and sedentary lifestyles to stress, pollution, and chronic diseases. However, by incorporating fresh juice into our daily routine; we can nourish our bodies with the essential nutrients they need to regenerate and renew themselves.

In this book, you will find a wealth of information and inspiration on how to use juicing to improve your health and well-being. You will discover how to select and store the best fruits and vegetables for juicing and learn which ones to avoid. You will also learn how to boost the nutritional value of your juice and how to find the right juicer for your needs.

The book covers a variety of health concerns, from managing diabetes and improving heart health to improving circulation, cleansing your system, and anti-aging. Each recipe is carefully crafted to address specific health concerns and promote optimal health and vitality.

Whether you are a seasoned juicer or just getting started, this book is designed to help you harness the power of fresh juice to improve your health and well-being in a natural, holistic way. So, let's get started on this exciting journey towards vibrant health and well-being!

Disclaimer: The information provided in this book is for educational and informational purposes only. The contents of this book have not been evaluated by the Food and Drug Administration and are not intended to diagnose, treat, or cure any medical condition. The information in this book should not be used as a substitute for professional medical advice, diagnosis, or treatment. It is always best to consult with a qualified healthcare provider for advice and information about your specific health concerns.

The author(s) of this book are not medical professionals and do not hold any certifications or licenses related to healthcare. The information contained in this book is based on the authors' personal experiences and research and is not intended to replace medical advice from a qualified healthcare provider.

The recipes in this book are intended to promote health and well-being, but individual results may vary. The author(s) of this book are not responsible for any adverse effects or consequences that may result from the use of the information or recipes contained in this book.

It is important to note that juicing can have potential side effects for certain individuals, such as those with certain medical conditions or who are taking certain medications. Before starting any new diet or juicing regimen, consult with a qualified healthcare provider to ensure it is safe and appropriate for you.

Note: The nutritional information provided is based on average values and may vary depending on the specific ingredients, size, and ripeness of the produce used.

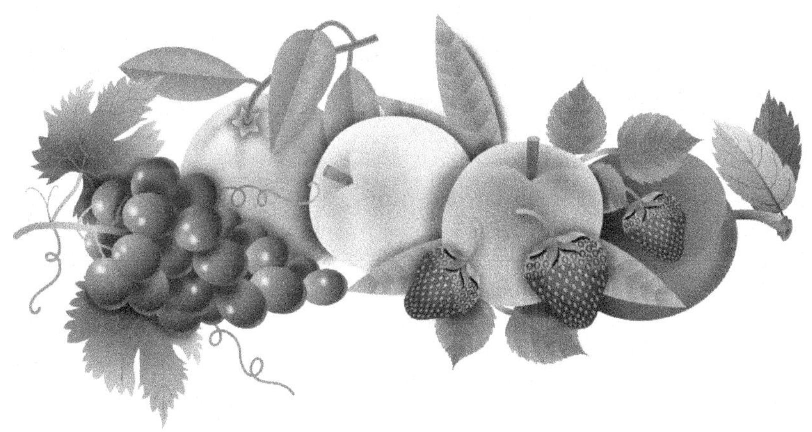

The Power of Juicing for Vibrant Health

"Let food be thy medicine and medicine be thy food." - Hippocrates.

Juicing is beneficial for your health and well-being in several ways:

1. **Provides essential nutrients:** Juicing allows you to consume a large quantity of fruits and vegetables in a single glass, providing you with essential vitamins, minerals, and phytonutrients that are vital for good health. Most people struggle to consume the recommended daily intake of fruits and vegetables, but juicing makes it easier to meet those goals.
2. **Enhances digestion:** Juicing breaks down fruits and vegetables into an easily digestible form, which allows your body to absorb nutrients more efficiently. It can also help stimulate digestive enzymes and promote regular bowel movements.
3. **Boosts immunity:** Fresh juices contain antioxidants and immune-boosting compounds that help strengthen your immune system and protect against diseases.
4. **Promotes weight loss:** Juicing can be an effective tool for weight loss, as it allows you to consume low-calorie, nutrient-dense foods that keep you feeling full and satisfied.
5. **Reduces inflammation:** Many fruits and vegetables have anti-inflammatory properties that can help reduce inflammation in the body, inflammation is one of the leading causes of chronic diseases such as arthritis, heart disease, and cancer.
6. **Detoxifies the body:** Juicing can help remove toxins from the body and promote healthy liver function. It can also help alkalize the body, which can help prevent chronic diseases.
7. **Improves energy levels:** Juicing provides your body with a quick burst of energy, as the nutrients are absorbed quickly into the bloodstream. Consuming this juice may aid in reducing fatigue and enhancing mental clarity.

Overall, juicing can be a valuable addition to a healthy lifestyle, providing a convenient and delicious way to boost your intake of essential nutrients and support your overall health and well-being.

The science behind juicing lies in the fact that it allows you to consume a concentrated dose of vitamins, minerals, and phytonutrients from fruits and vegetables in an easily digestible form. Juicing extracts the juice from fruits and vegetables, leaving behind the fibrous pulp, that allows your body to absorb the nutrients quickly and efficiently.

Juices are packed with antioxidants, vitamins, and minerals, that play essential roles in the body's functions. For example, antioxidants help protect cells from damage caused by free radicals, free radicals can contribute to aging and chronic diseases such as cancer, heart disease, and Alzheimer's disease.

Juicing can also help reduce inflammation in the body, inflammation is linked to several chronic diseases. Many fruits and vegetables, such as leafy greens, berries, and ginger, have anti-inflammatory properties that can help reduce inflammation.

Furthermore, juicing can provide a quick energy boost because the nutrients are absorbed quickly into the bloodstream. This can be especially helpful for athletes or anyone looking for a natural energy boost.

Finally, juicing can help support healthy digestion by providing a concentrated dose of fiber, enzymes, and other nutrients that can help regulate bowel movements and improve gut health.

While juicing can provide many health benefits, it is important to note that it's not a substitute for a healthy, balanced diet. Juices should be consumed in moderation, and it is important to include a variety of fruits and vegetables in your diet to ensure you are getting all the essential nutrients your body needs.

What juicer should I get?

There are several different types of juicers available on the market, and each has its pros and cons. Here is an overview of the most common types of juicers and how to choose the right one for your needs:

1. **Centrifugal juicers:** These are the most common and affordable type of juicers. They work by using a spinning blade to chop up fruits and vegetables and extract the juice through a mesh screen. They are fast and easy to use, but they can produce heat and oxygen that can degrade some of the nutrients in the juice. They also tend to produce more pulp and foam than other types of juicers.

2. **Masticating juicers:** Also known as slow juicers or cold-press juicers, these juicers work by crushing fruits and vegetables with a slow-rotating auger or gear. They produce less heat and oxygen than centrifugal juicers, which helps to preserve more of the nutrients in the juice. They also produce less foam and pulp and can extract more juice from leafy greens and other tough produce. They tend to be more expensive than centrifugal juicers, but they are more versatile and can be used to make other foods like nut butter and sorbet.

3. **Citrus juicers:** These juicers are designed specifically for citrus fruits like oranges, lemons, and grapefruits. They work by pressing the fruit against a reamer to extract the juice. They are simple and easy to use, but they are limited in their versatility.

4. **Twin-gear juicers:** These juicers use two gears that rotate together to crush and press fruits and vegetables to extract the juice. They are more efficient than other types of juicers and produce a higher yield of juice. In addition, they can be pricier and require more effort to clean.

When choosing a juicer, consider your budget, the types of produce you want to juice, and how often you plan to use it. If you are on a budget and want a fast and easy juicer, a centrifugal juicer may be the best choice for you. If you want to extract the most nutrients from your produce and are willing to invest in a higher-quality machine, a masticating juicer may be a better option. If you only plan to juice citrus fruits, a citrus juicer is the most practical choice. Finally, if you want the highest yield and are willing to spend more money, a twin-gear juicer may be the best choice.

Selecting your Produce

Buying and storing fresh produce properly is crucial to maintaining its quality and nutritional value. Here are some helpful tips for purchasing and storing fresh produce.:

Buying your produce:

- **Choose seasonal produce:** Seasonal produce is usually fresher, tastier, and more affordable than out-of-season produce.

- **Look for freshness:** Choose produce that is firm, brightly colored, and free from bruises or blemishes.

- **Smell the produce:** Fresh produce should have a mild, sweet aroma. If it smells sour or musty, it may be overripe or spoiled.

- **Check the labels:** Read the labels on packaged produce to ensure that they are free from preservatives and additives.

Storing your fruits and vegetables:

- **Store produce in the refrigerator:** Most fruits and vegetables should be stored in the refrigerator to maintain their freshness and quality.
- **Keep produce separate:** Fruits and vegetables give off ethylene gas, which can cause other produce to ripen and spoil faster. Keep them separate to avoid cross-contamination.
- **Store produce in the crisper drawer:** The crisper drawer in your refrigerator is designed to maintain humidity levels, which can help preserve the freshness of your produce.
- **Use airtight containers:** Use airtight containers to store chopped fruits and vegetables to prevent them from drying out or absorbing unwanted odors.
- **Do not wash produce until you're ready to use it:** Washing produce can cause it to spoil faster, so it's best to wait until you're ready to use it before washing.

By following these tips, you can ensure that your fresh produce stays fresh and delicious for as long as possible.

Best fruits and vegetables for juicing

- **Apples:** Apples are an excellent source of dietary fiber and vitamin C, both of which offer numerous health benefits. Additionally, regular consumption of apples has been associated with decreased cholesterol levels and reduced risk of heart disease.

- **Oranges:** Oranges are a good source of vitamin C and other antioxidants, which can help to boost the immune system and reduce the risk of chronic disease.

- **Pineapple:** Pineapple contains a digestive enzyme called bromelain, which can help to reduce inflammation and improve digestion.

- **Grapefruit:** Grapefruit is rich in vitamin C and has a low-calorie count. It is also known for its potential to lower cholesterol levels and to decrease the risk of heart disease.

- **Kiwi:** Kiwi provides a rich supply of vitamin C, fiber, and potassium, all of which contribute to good health. Furthermore, it can aid in digestion and alleviate inflammation.

- **Mango:** Mango is high in vitamin C and antioxidants; vitamin C and antioxidants have been shown to help boost the immune system and reduce the risk of chronic disease.

- **Papaya:** Papaya contains a digestive enzyme called papain, papain can help to improve digestion and reduce inflammation.

- **Berries (strawberries, blueberries, raspberries, etc.):** Berries are high in antioxidants, antioxidants have been shown to help protect against cell damage and reduce the risk of chronic disease.

- **Grapes:** Grapes are high in antioxidants and can help to improve blood flow and reduce the risk of heart disease.

- **Pomegranate:** Pomegranate is high in antioxidants and can help to improve blood flow and reduce the risk of chronic disease.

- **Watermelon:** Watermelon is low in calories and high in vitamin C and potassium. Vitamin C and potassium can also help to reduce inflammation and improve hydration.

- **Guava:** Guava is high in vitamin C and antioxidants.

- **Cherries:** Cherries are high in antioxidants and can help to reduce inflammation and improve sleep quality.

- **Cantaloupe:** Cantaloupe is high in vitamin C and antioxidants.

- **Lemon:** Lemon is high in vitamin C and can help to improve digestion and reduce inflammation.

- **Lime:** Lime is high in vitamin C and antioxidants.

- **Passion fruit:** Passion fruit is high in fiber and antioxidants, which can help to improve digestion and reduce the risk of chronic disease.

- **Persimmon:** Persimmon is high in vitamin C and fiber, vitamin C and fiber can help to improve digestion and reduce the risk of chronic disease.

- **Starfruit:** Starfruit is a nutrient-dense fruit that is low in calories but high in vitamin C and fiber. It is also known to aid in digestion and reduce inflammation.

- **Cranberries:** Cranberries are high in antioxidants and can help to reduce inflammation and improve urinary tract health.

- **Blackberries:** Blackberries are high in antioxidants and can help to improve brain function and reduce inflammation.

- **Raspberries:** Raspberries are high in antioxidants and can help to reduce inflammation and improve heart health.

- **Gooseberries:** Gooseberries are high in vitamin C and antioxidants.

- **Tangerines:** Tangerines are a good source of vitamin C and can help to improve skin health and reduce the risk of chronic disease.

- **Apricots:** Apricots are high in vitamin C and antioxidants.

- **Carrots:** high in beta-carotene and vitamin A, which promotes healthy vision and skin.

- **Spinach:** contains iron, folate, and vitamin K, which helps with blood clotting and bone health.

- **Kale:** high in vitamin C, antioxidants, and calcium, which may lower the risk of heart disease and osteoporosis.

- **Beets:** high in nitrates, which help improve blood flow and lower blood pressure.

- **Cucumber:** high in water content and low in calories, which helps with hydration and weight loss.

- **Celery:** contains potassium and antioxidants, potassium and antioxidants have been shown to help with blood pressure and inflammation.

- **Broccoli:** high in vitamin C, vitamin K, and fiber, which supports immunity and digestion.

- **Ginger:** has anti-inflammatory properties and may help with nausea and digestion.

- **Parsley:** high in vitamin K and antioxidants, which may improve bone health and protect against chronic diseases.

- **Fennel:** contains fiber and antioxidants, fiber and antioxidants may help with digestion and inflammation.

- **Swiss chard:** contains vitamin K, magnesium, and antioxidants, which may help with bone health and lower the risk of chronic diseases.

- **Tomatoes:** high in lycopene, which may help protect against cancer and heart disease.

- **Garlic:** contains sulfur compounds, which may lower cholesterol and blood pressure.

- **Bell peppers:** high in vitamin C and antioxidants, which may boost immunity and reduce the risk of chronic diseases.

- **Wheatgrass:** high in chlorophyll and antioxidants, which may improve digestion and detoxification.

- **Radish:** high in vitamin C and antioxidants, which may help with immunity and inflammation.

- **Sweet potato:** high in beta-carotene, vitamin C, and fiber, which may help with digestion and promote healthy skin.

- **Spinach:** high in iron, folate, and vitamin K, which helps with blood clotting and bone health.

- **Green cabbage:** contains vitamin K and antioxidants, which may help with bone health and reduce inflammation.

- **Pumpkin:** high in beta-carotene, which may promote healthy skin and eyes.

- **Brussels sprouts:** high in vitamin C and fiber, which may improve digestion and reduce inflammation.

- **Artichoke:** contains fiber and antioxidants, which may help with digestion and liver function.

- **Zucchini:** low in calories and high in water content, which helps with hydration and weight loss.

- **Cauliflower:** high in vitamin C and antioxidants, which may reduce inflammation and lower the risk of chronic diseases.

- **Asparagus:** contains fiber and antioxidants, which may help with digestion and reduce inflammation.

By incorporating these fruits and vegetables into your juice recipes, you can create delicious and nutritious blends that promote health and wellness.

What fruits and vegetable to avoid juicing

While most fruits and vegetables are great for juicing, there are some that you may want to avoid or use in moderation, depending on your specific health needs. Here are a few examples:

- **Bananas:** Bananas are not typically used in juicing because they are soft and do not yield much juice. However, you can still incorporate them into your juice by blending them with other fruits and vegetables.

- **Avocado:** Avocado is another fruit that is not typically used in juicing because it is high in fat and does not yield much juice. However, you can still incorporate it into your juice by blending it with other ingredients to create a smoothie.

- **Rhubarb:** While rhubarb is a great source of vitamins and minerals, it is not typically used in juicing because it is high in oxalic acid, which can be harmful in large quantities. If you do choose to use rhubarb in your juice, be sure to use it in small amounts.

- **Spinach:** Spinach is a popular ingredient in juicing, but it should be used in moderation because it contains oxalic acid, which can be harmful in large quantities. If you do use spinach in your juice, try mixing it with other leafy greens to dilute its oxalic acid content.

- **Grapefruit:** Grapefruit can interfere with certain medications, so if you are taking any medications, it is best to avoid using grapefruit in your juice.

Overall, it is important to use a variety of fruits and vegetables in your juice to ensure that you are getting a wide range of nutrients. If there are certain fruits or vegetables that you need to avoid or use in moderation, try experimenting with different combinations of ingredients to find what works best for you.

Boost your Juice

1. **Spirulina powder** - high in protein, antioxidants, and nutrients
2. **Wheatgrass powder** - detoxifying and alkalizing properties, rich in vitamins and minerals
3. **Matcha powder** - high in antioxidants and can boost metabolism
4. **Turmeric powder** - anti-inflammatory and can help with digestion and joint pain
5. **Ashwagandha powder** - adaptogenic herb that can help with stress and anxiety
6. **Chlorella powder** - detoxifying and immune-boosting properties
7. **Acai berry powder** - high in antioxidants and can help with cardiovascular health
8. **Baobab powder** - high in vitamin C and can help with digestion and immunity
9. **Maca powder** - adaptogenic herb that can help with energy and hormone balance
10. **Cacao powder** - high in antioxidants and can improve mood and cognitive function
11. **Ginger powder** - anti-inflammatory and can help with digestion and nausea
12. **Moringa powder** - high in vitamins and minerals and can help with inflammation and blood sugar control
13. **Beetroot powder** - high in nitrates and can help with blood pressure and exercise performance
14. **Pumpkin seed powder** - high in protein and can help with prostate health
15. **Hemp protein powder** - high in protein and omega-3 fatty acids
16. **Flaxseed powder** - high in fiber and omega-3 fatty acids, can help with heart health and digestion
17. **Camu camu powder** - high in vitamin C and can help with immune function and skin health
18. **Goji berry powder** - high in antioxidants and can help with eye health and immunity
19. **Reishi mushroom powder** - adaptogenic herb that can help with immune function and stress
20. **Lion's mane mushroom powder** - can improve cognitive function and brain health

Please note that some of these powders may interact with certain medications or medical conditions, so it is important to consult with a healthcare professional before adding them to your diet.

Vitamins and Minerals in Juicing

- **Vitamin A -** Vitamin A is crucial for maintaining healthy vision, skin, and immune system function. It is important to incorporate foods rich in vitamin A into your diet to ensure that you're meeting your daily requirements. Some examples of fruits and vegetables high in vitamin A include carrots, sweet potatoes, kale, spinach, and cantaloupe.

- **Vitamin C -** Vitamin C is an antioxidant that helps protect cells from damage and is important for skin health, immune function, and iron absorption. Fruits and vegetables high in vitamin C include oranges, grapefruits, lemons, strawberries, kiwis, bell peppers, and broccoli.

- **Vitamin E -** Vitamin E is also an antioxidant and helps protect cells from damage. It is important for immune function, skin health, and may have a role in protecting against heart disease. Fruits and vegetables high in vitamin E include almonds, spinach, sweet potatoes, avocados, and butternut squash.

- **Vitamin K -** Vitamin K plays a crucial role in blood clotting and bone health maintenance. Foods that are high in vitamin K include kale, spinach, broccoli, asparagus, and Brussels sprouts.

- **Vitamin B1 (Thiamine) -** Vitamin B1 is important for energy metabolism and proper functioning of the nervous system. Fruits and vegetables high in vitamin B1 include asparagus, spinach, peas, oranges, and cantaloupe.

- **Vitamin B2 (Riboflavin) -** Vitamin B2 is important for energy metabolism and the production of red blood cells. Fruits and vegetables high in vitamin B2 include spinach, mushrooms, almonds, and avocados.

- **Vitamin B3 (Niacin) -** Vitamin B3 is important for energy metabolism and the proper functioning of the nervous system. Fruits and vegetables high in vitamin B3 include mushrooms, asparagus, sweet potatoes, and avocados.

- **Vitamin B6 -** Vitamin B6 is important for protein metabolism, the production of red blood cells, and the proper functioning of the nervous system. Fruits and vegetables high in vitamin B6 include bananas, sweet potatoes, spinach, and bell peppers.

- **Vitamin B9 (Folate) -** Vitamin B9, also known as folate, plays a crucial role in the production of new cells, including red blood cells, and is particularly important for pregnant women, as it can help prevent birth defects. To ensure adequate intake of this essential vitamin, incorporating folate-rich fruits and vegetables such as spinach, broccoli, asparagus, and avocado into your diet is recommended.

- **Vitamin B12 -** Vitamin B12 is important to produce red blood cells and the proper functioning of the nervous system. It is found mainly in animal products, but can also be found in fortified plant-based milks and nutritional yeast.

- **Calcium -** Calcium is important for building and maintaining strong bones and teeth, muscle function, and nerve transmission. Fruits and vegetables high in calcium include kale, spinach, broccoli, and oranges.

- **Iron -** Iron is important to produce hemoglobin, which carries oxygen in the blood. Fruits and vegetables high in iron include spinach, kale, lentils, and tofu.

- **Magnesium -** Magnesium is important for muscle and nerve function and plays a role in energy metabolism and bone health. Fruits and vegetables high in magnesium include spinach, almonds, avocado, and bananas.

- **Potassium -** Potassium is important for maintaining proper fluid balance in the body and is also involved in nerve and muscle function. Fruits and vegetables high in potassium include bananas, oranges, spinach, and sweet potatoes.

- **Zinc -** Zinc is important for immune function, wound healing, and cell growth and division. Fruits and vegetables high in zinc include spinach, mushrooms, avocado, and asparagus.

Notes:

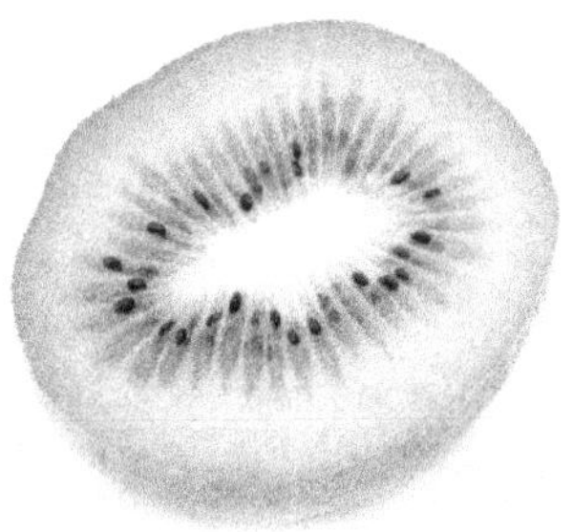

Preventing and Living with Diabetes

"Juices are like dynamite — a quick explosive burst of goodness, that requires only minutes to consume but delivers hours of fuel to the body." - Jay Kordich

Gaining an understanding of the connection between diet and diabetes.

Diabetes is a persistent health condition arising from inadequate insulin production or ineffective utilization of the insulin produced by the body. Insulin is a hormone that plays a crucial role in maintaining healthy blood sugar levels. There are two primary types of diabetes: type 1, which is caused by an autoimmune response that damages insulin-producing cells in the pancreas, and type 2, which results from a combination of genetic and lifestyle factors such as physical inactivity and obesity. It is essential to manage diabetes effectively to prevent complications and maintain overall health.

Diet plays a crucial role in the management and prevention of type 2 diabetes, as well as in the treatment of type 1 diabetes. When we eat, our body breaks down the carbohydrates in our food into glucose, which is then absorbed into the bloodstream and used for energy. Insulin helps to regulate the amount of glucose in the blood by signaling to cells to take up glucose and use it for energy or store it for later use. In people with diabetes, this process is disrupted, leading to high blood sugar levels that can cause a range of health problems over time.

A healthy diet for diabetes management typically includes a balance of carbohydrates, proteins, and fats, as well as plenty of fruits, vegetables, and whole grains. The goal is to choose foods that are high in fiber and nutrients but low in refined carbohydrates and added sugars, which can cause blood sugar spikes.

In addition to eating a healthy diet, people with diabetes may also need to monitor their blood sugar levels, take medications or insulin as prescribed by their healthcare provider, and engage in regular physical activity to help manage their condition. By working with their healthcare team and making lifestyle changes, people with diabetes can live healthy, active lives and reduce their risk of long-term complications such as nerve damage, kidney disease, and cardiovascular disease.

Do's:

- Choose low-glycemic index fruits and vegetables, such as leafy greens, berries, and citrus fruits.
- Include protein and healthy fats in your juice to help slow down the absorption of sugar into the bloodstream.
- Check your blood sugar levels regularly and adjust your juice recipes accordingly.
- Consider incorporating ginger and cinnamon into your juice recipes, as they can help regulate blood sugar levels.
- It is always important to seek guidance from your healthcare provider before making significant changes to your diet.

Don'ts:

- Avoid juicing high-glycemic index fruits and vegetables, such as pineapple, watermelon, and beets, in large quantities.
- Avoid adding sweeteners to your juice, such as honey or maple syrup, as they can raise blood sugar levels.
- Don't rely solely on juice as a meal replacement. It's essential to have a balanced diet that includes a variety of whole foods.

Warnings and advice:

- Drinking too much juice can lead to weight gain; weight gain can increase your risk of developing diabetes or exacerbate existing diabetes.
- Juicing can cause a rapid increase in blood sugar levels, which can be dangerous for people with diabetes. Monitor your blood sugar levels and adjust your intake accordingly.
- It's important to include fiber in your diet to help slow down the absorption of sugar into the bloodstream. Consider adding fiber-rich ingredients such as chia seeds or ground flaxseed to your juice recipes.

Low glycaemic index foods your Diabetes Juice:

- **Spinach:** This leafy green vegetable is low in carbohydrates and has a glycemic index of only 15, making spinach an excellent choice for juicing.

- **Kale:** Another nutrient-rich leafy green vegetable, kale has a glycemic index of 32 and can add a lot of nutritional value to your juice.

- **Cucumber:** Cucumbers are low in carbohydrates and have a glycemic index of 15, making cucumber a refreshing addition to your juice.

- **Broccoli:** Broccoli is high in fiber and has a glycemic index of only 10, making broccoli a great choice for juicing.

- **Green beans:** green beans are low in carbohydrates and have a glycemic index of only 15, making green beans a good choice for people with diabetes.

- **Berries:** Many types of berries, such as strawberries, raspberries, and blueberries, have a low glycemic index and are packed with antioxidants and other nutrients.

- **Tomatoes:** Tomatoes are low in carbohydrates and have a glycemic index of only 15, making tomatoes a good choice for juicing.

- **Carrots:** Carrots are higher in carbohydrates than some of the other vegetables on this list, but they still have a relatively low glycemic index of 35.

- **Bell peppers:** Bell peppers are low in carbohydrates and have a glycemic index of only 15, making bell peppers a colorful and nutritious addition to your juice.

- **Citrus fruits:** Many types of citrus fruits, such as oranges and grapefruits, have a low glycemic index and can add a burst of flavor and vitamin C to your juice.

Remember to always check with your healthcare provider before adding new foods or drinks to your diet, especially if you have diabetes or other health conditions.

Boost your Diabetes Juice

- **Cinnamon powder:** Cinnamon has been shown to lower blood sugar levels by improving insulin sensitivity. Adding cinnamon powder to your juice may help regulate blood sugar levels.

- **Gymnema Sylvestre powder**: This herb has been used for centuries in Ayurvedic medicine to manage blood sugar levels. Gymnema Sylvestre powder may improve glucose uptake by cells, reducing blood sugar levels.

- **Fenugreek powder:** Fenugreek is another herb that has been shown to help lower blood sugar levels. It may also improve insulin sensitivity and reduce insulin resistance.

- **Amla powder:** Amla, or Indian gooseberry, is a rich source of vitamin C and antioxidants. It may help improve glucose metabolism and reduce the risk of diabetic complications.

- **Turmeric powder:** Turmeric contains a compound called curcumin, which has anti-inflammatory properties and may help improve insulin sensitivity.

- **Moringa powder:** Moringa powder is derived from a plant native to India, which has been utilized for centuries in Ayurvedic medicine. It is believed to have potential in improving insulin sensitivity and lowering blood sugar levels.

- **Ginger powder:** Ginger has anti-inflammatory properties and may help improve insulin sensitivity. It may also reduce the risk of diabetic complications by improving blood lipid levels.

It is important to note that adding these to your juice should not replace any medications or medical advice given by your healthcare provider.

Spinach-Cucumber-Kale Juice

Ingredients:

2 cups spinach
1 cucumber
2 kale leaves

Instructions:

Wash all the ingredients thoroughly.
Chop the cucumber and kale into pieces that can fit into your juicer.
Put the ingredients into the juicer and extract the juice.
Pour the juice into a glass and enjoy!

Benefits:

This juice is packed with a variety of vitamins, minerals, and antioxidants that can provide many health benefits. Spinach is a great source of iron, calcium, and vitamins A and C, which can help support healthy bones, skin, and immunity. Cucumbers contain water, fiber, and antioxidants, which can help keep you hydrated, promote digestion, and reduce inflammation. Kale is a nutrient-dense leafy green that contains vitamins K, A, and C, as well as minerals like calcium, iron, and potassium, which can help support healthy bones, vision, and immunity.

Nutritional information:

Serving size: 1 glass (about 12 ounces)
Calories: 46
Total fat: 0.5g
Saturated fat: 0.1g
Cholesterol: 0mg
Sodium: 46mg
Total carbohydrates: 10g
Total sugars: 3.3g
Protein: 3g

Green Juice

Ingredients:

2 cups spinach
1/2 cucumber
2 celery stalks
1/2 green apple
1/2 lemon, peeled
1-inch piece of ginger

Instructions:

Wash all the ingredients thoroughly.
Chop the cucumber, celery, apple, and ginger into small pieces.
Put the ingredients into the juicer and extract the juice.
Pour the juice into a glass and enjoy!

Benefits:

Spinach is a low-glycemic index vegetable that helps regulate blood sugar levels.
Cucumber is rich in fiber and helps control blood sugar levels.
Celery is rich in anti-inflammatory properties that can aid in reducing blood sugar levels.
Green apple is low in sugar and helps regulate blood sugar levels.
Lemon is a good source of vitamin C and can help improve insulin sensitivity.
Ginger has anti-inflammatory properties and can help improve insulin sensitivity.

Nutritional Information:

Calories: 78
Carbohydrates: 19g
Protein: 3g
Fat: 1g
Sugar: 11g
Sodium: 102mg

Carrot-Apple-Ginger Juice

Ingredients:

4 large carrots
2 green apples
1-inch piece of ginger root

Instructions:

Wash the carrots, apples, and ginger root thoroughly.
Chop the carrots and apples into pieces small enough to fit in your juicer.
Peel the ginger root and cut it into small pieces.
Put the ingredients into the juicer and extract the juice.
Pour the juice into a glass and enjoy!

Benefits:

Carrots are rich in beta-carotene, which is converted to vitamin A in the body and supports healthy vision and immune function.
Apples are a good source of fiber and contain antioxidants that protect against oxidative damage.
Ginger has anti-inflammatory properties and can help alleviate nausea and indigestion.

Nutritional Information:

Calories: 154
Fat: 0.7g
Protein: 2.3g
Carbohydrates: 39.4g
Sugar: 23.5g
Sodium: 118mg

Carrot and Beet Juice

Ingredients:

3 carrots
1 small beet
1/2 lemon, peeled
1-inch piece of ginger

Instructions:

Wash all the ingredients thoroughly.
Chop the carrots and beet into small pieces.
Put the ingredients into the juicer and extract the juice.
Pour the juice into a glass and enjoy!

Benefits:

Carrots are rich in beta-carotene, which can help improve insulin sensitivity.
Beets are an excellent source of nitrates, which the body converts into nitric oxide. This has been shown to increase blood flow and reduce blood pressure, making them a beneficial part of any diet.
Lemon is a good source of vitamin C and can help improve insulin resistance.
Ginger has anti-inflammatory properties and can help prevent diabetes-related complications.

Nutritional Information:

Calories: 118
Carbohydrates: 28g
Protein: 3g
Fat: 1g
Sugar: 16g
Sodium: 115mg

Bitter Gourd and Spinach Juice

Ingredients:

1 medium-sized bitter gourd, sliced
2 cups spinach leaves
1/2 green apple
1/2 lemon, peeled

Instructions:

Wash all the ingredients thoroughly.
Chop the bitter gourd into small pieces.
Remove the core and seeds of the apple and cut it into small pieces.
Put the ingredients into the juicer and extract the juice.
Pour the juice into a glass and enjoy!

Benefits:

Bitter gourd can help regulate blood sugar levels and improve insulin sensitivity.
Spinach is rich in antioxidants and can help prevent diabetes-related complications.
Green apple is low in sugar and can help improve digestion.
Lemon is a good source of vitamin C and can help improve insulin resistance.

Nutritional Information:

Calories: 97
Carbohydrates: 24g
Protein: 3g
Fat: 1g
Sugar: 10g
Sodium: 67mg

Spinach and Kale Juice

Ingredients:

2 cups spinach
2 cups kale
2 green apples, cored and chopped
1 cucumber
1 lemon, peeled

Instructions:

Wash all the ingredients thoroughly.
Chop the apples and cucumber into small pieces.
Put the ingredients into the juicer and extract the juice.
Pour the juice into a glass and enjoy!

Benefits:

Spinach and kale are low in calories and high in fiber, which can help regulate blood sugar levels.
Green apples are rich in polyphenols, which can help improve insulin sensitivity.
Cucumber is high in water and can help reduce blood sugar levels.

Nutritional Information:

Calories: 194
Carbohydrates: 49g
Protein: 7g
Fat: 1g
Sugar: 26g
Sodium: 99mg

Carrot and Cucumber Juice

Ingredients:

4 medium carrots
1 medium cucumber
1/2 lemon, peeled
1-inch piece of fresh ginger, peeled

Instructions:

Wash all the ingredients thoroughly.
Chop the carrots and cucumber into small pieces.
Put the ingredients into the juicer and extract the juice.
Pour the juice into a glass and enjoy!

Benefits:

Carrots are high in beta-carotene, which can help improve insulin sensitivity.
Cucumbers are low in calories and can help regulate blood sugar levels.
Ginger contains anti-inflammatory properties that can aid in enhancing digestion.

Nutritional Information:

Calories: 121
Carbohydrates: 28g
Protein: 3g
Fat: 1g
Sugar: 16g
Sodium: 118mg

Tomato-Carrot-Celery Juice

Ingredients:

4 large tomatoes
4 large carrots
4 stalks of celery

Instructions:

Wash the tomatoes, carrots, and celery thoroughly.
Chop the tomatoes into quarters, and the carrots and celery into pieces small enough to fit in your juicer.
Put the ingredients into the juicer and extract the juice.
Pour the juice into a glass and enjoy!

Benefits:

Tomatoes are rich in lycopene, an antioxidant that helps protect against certain cancers.
Carrots are a good source of beta-carotene, which is converted to vitamin A in the body and supports healthy vision and immune function.
Celery is low in calories and high in fiber, which can help support healthy digestion.

Nutritional Information:

Calories: 141
Fat: 0.7g
Protein: 5.2g
Carbohydrates: 31.9g
Sugar: 19.5g
Sodium: 223mg

Beetroot-Carrot-Lemon Juice

Ingredients:

2 medium beetroots
4 large carrots
1/2 lemon

Instructions:

Wash the beetroots, carrots, and lemon thoroughly.
Peel the beetroots and carrots, and chop them into pieces small enough to fit in your juicer.
Peel the lemon and cut in half, remove any seeds.
Put the ingredients into the juicer and extract the juice.
Pour the juice into a glass and enjoy!

Benefits:

Beetroots are rich in nitrates, which can help improve blood flow and regulate blood sugar levels.
Carrots are a good source of beta-carotene, which supports healthy vision and immune function.
Lemons are high in vitamin C, an antioxidant that helps protect against cellular damage and supports immune function.

Nutritional Information:

Calories: 156
Fat: 0.7g
Protein: 4.3g
Carbohydrates: 36.4g
Sugar: 20.9g
Sodium: 215mg

Green Apple-Cucumber-Kale Juice

Ingredients:

2 medium green apples
1 large cucumber
2 cups of kale leaves

Instructions:

Wash the green apples, cucumber, and kale thoroughly.
Core the apples and chop them into pieces small enough to fit in your juicer.
Cut the cucumber into pieces small enough to fit in your juicer.
Remove the kale leaves from their stems.
Put all the ingredients into the juicer and extract the juice.
Pour the juice into a glass and enjoy!

Benefits:

Green apples are high in fiber and antioxidants, which can help regulate blood sugar levels and reduce inflammation.
Cucumbers are low in calories and high in water content, which can help promote hydration and weight management.
Kale is a nutrient-dense leafy green that is high in vitamins A, C, and K, as well as minerals like calcium and potassium. These nutrients can support overall health and immune function.

Nutritional Information:

Calories: 173
Fat: 1.1g
Protein: 6.8g
Carbohydrates: 39.9g
Sugar: 27.6g
Sodium: 86mg

Managing diabetes through juicing

Juicing can be a helpful tool for managing diabetes, but it should be approached with caution and in consultation with a healthcare provider. Here are some tips for using juicing as part of a healthy lifestyle for diabetes management:

- **Choose low-glycemic fruits and vegetables:** Fruits and vegetables with a low glycemic index (GI) are less likely to cause spikes in blood sugar levels. Some examples are leafy greens, berries, and citrus fruits.
- **Use a variety of fruits and vegetables:** By using a mix of different fruits and vegetables, you can ensure that you are getting a wide range of vitamins, minerals, and antioxidants that can support overall health and help manage diabetes.
- **Avoid added sugars:** Avoid adding sugar or other sweeteners to your juices, as these can cause blood sugar spikes.
- **Consider adding protein:** Protein can help slow the absorption of carbohydrates and help keep blood sugar levels more stable. Consider adding sources of protein such as Greek yogurt, nuts, or seeds to your juices.
- **Drink juices in moderation:** While juices can be a healthy addition to a diabetes management plan, they should be consumed in moderation as they can still contain a significant amount of carbohydrates.

In addition to juicing, there are several other lifestyle habits that can help manage diabetes, including:

- **Eating a balanced diet:** As mentioned earlier, a balanced diet that is rich in whole foods, fiber, and low in refined carbohydrates and added sugars can help manage diabetes.
- **Engaging in regular physical activity:** Regular exercise can help improve insulin sensitivity and help manage blood sugar levels.
- **Monitoring blood sugar levels:** It's important to regularly monitor blood sugar levels and to work with a healthcare provider to adjust medications or lifestyle habits as needed.
- **Managing stress:** Stress can cause blood sugar levels to rise, so it's important to find ways to manage stress, such as through mindfulness, yoga, or other stress-reducing techniques.

By incorporating healthy lifestyle habits, including juicing, people with diabetes can better manage their condition and reduce their risk of long-term complications.

In conclusion, diabetes is a serious and chronic health condition that affects millions of people around the world. It can lead to a range of complications, such as heart disease, kidney disease, nerve damage, and vision problems. However, by making lifestyle changes and working with healthcare providers to manage their condition, people with diabetes can live healthy, active lives and reduce their risk of long-term complications.

One of the most important ways to manage and prevent diabetes is through diet. By choosing foods that are high in fiber and nutrients but low in refined carbohydrates and added sugars, people with diabetes can help regulate their blood sugar levels and reduce their risk of health problems. This means eating plenty of fruits, vegetables, whole grains, lean proteins, and healthy fats.

Juicing can be a convenient and tasty way to incorporate more fruits and vegetables into your diet. However, it's important to choose low-glycemic index ingredients, such as leafy greens, berries, and citrus fruits, and to avoid adding sweeteners like honey or maple syrup that can raise blood sugar levels. Adding protein and healthy fats to your juice can help slow down the absorption of sugar into the bloodstream. Incorporating ginger and cinnamon can help regulate blood sugar levels.

In addition to making dietary changes, people with diabetes may need to monitor their blood sugar levels regularly and take medications or insulin as prescribed by their healthcare provider. Engaging in regular physical activity can also help manage diabetes by improving insulin sensitivity and blood sugar control.

It's important to work closely with a healthcare provider to manage diabetes effectively. This may involve regular check-ups, blood tests, and adjustments to medication or insulin doses. By working with their healthcare team and making lifestyle changes, people with diabetes can live healthy, active lives and reduce their risk of long-term complications.

Note: These recipes are not intended to treat or cure any medical condition. Please consult with your healthcare provider before making any significant changes to your diet.

Notes:

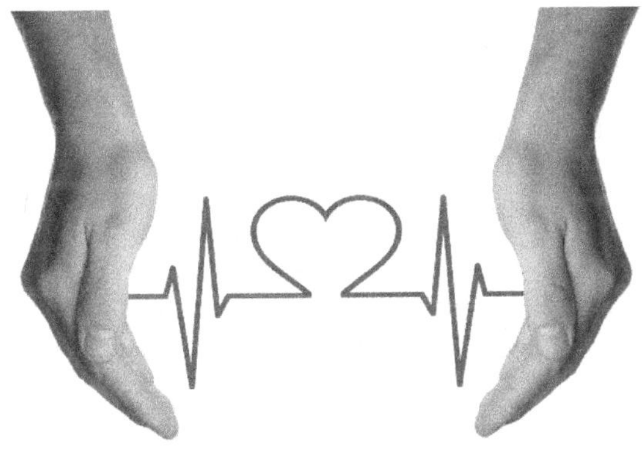

Heart Health

"The doctor of the future will give no medication, but will interest his patients in the care of the human frame, diet and in the cause and prevention of disease." - Thomas A. Edison

The importance of a healthy heart

Heart disease is a leading cause of death worldwide, and it is essential to take steps to reduce the risk of developing this condition. The heart is responsible for pumping blood throughout the body, and when it is not working correctly, it can lead to a range of health problems, including heart attacks, strokes, and heart failure. Here are some reasons why heart health is so important and steps you can take to reduce the risk of heart disease:

- **Heart health is critical for overall health:** The heart is responsible for pumping blood and oxygen to all parts of the body, so when it is not working correctly, it can impact many different systems and organs.

- **Heart disease is preventable:** Many risk factors for heart disease, such as high blood pressure, smoking, and a poor diet, are modifiable. By making lifestyle changes, such as eating a healthy diet, getting regular exercise, and quitting smoking, you can significantly reduce your risk of developing heart disease.

- **Lifestyle changes can improve heart health:** Even if you already have heart disease or are at risk of developing it, lifestyle changes can help improve heart health and reduce the risk of complications. For example, regular exercise can help strengthen the heart and reduce blood pressure, while a heart-healthy diet can help lower cholesterol levels.

- **Early detection and treatment are essential:** Regular check-ups with a healthcare provider can help identify risk factors for heart disease and detect early signs of heart problems. Early detection and treatment can help prevent or delay the progression of heart disease and improve outcomes.

By making lifestyle changes to improve heart health, such as eating a healthy diet, getting regular exercise, and managing stress, you can significantly reduce your risk of developing heart disease and improve your overall health and well-being.

Do's:

- Choose vegetables and fruits that are high in antioxidants, such as blueberries, strawberries, spinach, and kale.
- Use fresh vegetables and fruits whenever possible.
- Incorporate heart-healthy fats into your juices, such as avocados and nuts.
- Consider adding ginger or turmeric to your juices, ginger and turmeric have been shown to have anti-inflammatory properties.
- Drink your juice immediately after making it to maximize its nutritional value.

Don'ts:

- Avoid using fruits and vegetables that are high in sugar, such as grapes and bananas, in large quantities.
- Do not add extra sugar or sweeteners to your juice.
- Avoid using too much salt or sodium-rich vegetables, such as celery, which can increase blood pressure.

Warnings:

- Consult with your doctor before making significant changes to your diet or starting a juicing regimen, particularly if you have a heart condition or are on medication.
- Juicing should not be a substitute for a balanced and varied diet that includes whole foods and other sources of nutrients.
- Drinking too much juice can lead to an excessive intake of calories and sugar, which can contribute to weight gain and other health problems.

Advice:

- If you have a history of heart disease or high cholesterol, consider adding heart-healthy supplements to your juice, such as omega-3 fatty acids or plant sterols.
- Be mindful of portion sizes and calorie intake, as excessive calorie consumption can lead to weight gain and other health problems.
- Monitor your blood sugar and blood pressure levels closely when incorporating juicing into your diet, particularly if you have diabetes or high blood pressure.

Foods for your Heart Health Juice

- **Beets:** Beets are rich in nitrates, which help to relax and widen blood vessels, resulting in lower blood pressure and improved blood flow.

- **Kale:** Kale is packed with antioxidants and anti-inflammatory compounds that help protect the heart from damage.

- **Spinach:** Spinach is a good source of magnesium, which helps regulate blood pressure and maintain healthy heart function.

- **Carrots:** Carrots are high in beta-carotene, which has been linked to a lower risk of heart disease.

- **Apples:** Apples are high in fiber and antioxidants, which help to reduce cholesterol levels and lower the risk of heart disease.

- **Blueberries:** Blueberries are packed with anthocyanins, which help to reduce inflammation and improve circulation.

- **Pomegranates:** Pomegranates are rich in polyphenols, which have been shown to reduce the risk of heart disease by improving blood flow and reducing inflammation.

- **Tomatoes:** Tomatoes are rich in lycopene, which has been linked to a reduced risk of heart disease.

- **Ginger:** Ginger has anti-inflammatory properties that can help reduce inflammation and improve heart health.

- **Garlic:** Garlic contains allicin, a compound that has been shown to lower cholesterol levels and reduce the risk of heart disease.

Boost your Heart Health Juice

- **Beetroot Powder** - Beetroot powder contains nitrates that help to widen blood vessels and lower blood pressure.

- **Cacao Powder** - Cacao powder is rich in flavonoids, which have been shown to help lower blood pressure, reduce inflammation, and improve overall heart health.

- **Garlic Powder** - Garlic powder contains compounds that help to lower blood pressure, reduce inflammation, and improve cholesterol levels.

- **Green Tea Powder** - Green tea powder is rich in catechins, which help to improve blood flow and lower cholesterol levels.

- **Hawthorn Berry Powder** - Hawthorn berry powder is a traditional remedy for heart health and has been shown to help improve blood pressure and circulation.

- **Hibiscus Powder** - Hibiscus powder is rich in antioxidants that help to lower blood pressure and reduce inflammation.

- **Turmeric Powder** - Turmeric powder contains curcumin, a compound that helps to reduce inflammation and improve heart health by lowering cholesterol levels.

- **Wheatgrass Powder** - Wheatgrass powder is rich in chlorophyll, which helps to improve blood flow and oxygenation, and may also help to lower cholesterol levels.

It's important to note that these should not be used as a substitute for medical treatment, and individuals with pre-existing medical conditions should consult their doctor before using any supplements.

Beet Juice

Ingredients:

2 beets
2 carrots
1 orange
1-inch piece of ginger

Instructions:

Wash all the ingredients thoroughly.
Peel the beetroots and carrots, and chop them into small pieces.
Peel the orange and separate the segments.
Put the ingredients into the juicer and extract the juice.
Pour the juice into a glass and enjoy!

Benefits:

Beetroot contains high levels of nitrates that can help reduce blood
pressure and improve blood circulation.
Carrots are a good source of vitamin A and can help improve heart health.
Orange is a good source of vitamin C and can help improve blood
pressure.
Ginger has anti-inflammatory properties and can help improve heart health.

Nutritional Information:

Calories: 159
Carbohydrates: 38g
Protein: 4g
Fat: 1g
Sugar: 23g
Sodium: 164mg

Green Juice

Ingredients:

2 cups kale
1 cucumber
2 celery stalks
1/2 green apple
1/2 lemon, peeled
1-inch piece of ginger

Instructions:

Wash all the ingredients thoroughly.
Chop the cucumber, celery, and apple into small pieces.
Put the ingredients into the juicer and extract the juice.
Pour the juice into a glass and enjoy!

Benefits:

Kale is rich in vitamins and minerals that can help improve heart health.
Cucumber is a good source of fiber and can help lower blood pressure.
Celery has anti-inflammatory properties and can help improve heart health.
Green apple is low in sugar and can help regulate blood pressure.
Lemon is a good source of vitamin C and can help improve cholesterol levels.
Ginger has anti-inflammatory properties and can help improve heart health.

Nutritional Information:

Calories: 81
Carbohydrates: 19g
Protein: 3g
Fat: 1g
Sugar: 10g
Sodium: 112mg

Watermelon and Mint Juice

Ingredients:

4 cups watermelon, chopped
1/4 cup fresh mint leaves
1/2 lemon, peeled

Instructions:

Wash all the ingredients thoroughly.
Chop the watermelon into small pieces.
Add the watermelon and mint to your juicer and extract the juice.
Squeeze the lemon juice into the juice and stir well.
Pour the juice into a glass and enjoy!

Benefits:

Watermelon is high in lycopene, which can help improve heart health.
Mint has anti-inflammatory properties and can help improve digestion.
Lemon is a good source of vitamin C and can help improve cholesterol
levels.

Nutritional Information:

Calories: 149
Carbohydrates: 38g
Protein: 3g
Fat: 1g
Sugar: 29g
Sodium: 6mg

Blueberry and Kale Juice

Ingredients:

1 cup blueberries
1 cup kale
1/2 lemon, peeled
1-inch piece of ginger

Instructions:

Wash all the ingredients thoroughly.
Put the ingredients into the juicer and extract the juice.
Pour the juice into a glass and enjoy!

Benefits:

Blueberries are rich in antioxidants, which can help reduce inflammation and improve heart health.
Kale is a good source of vitamins and minerals, which can help strengthen the heart and reduce the risk of heart disease.
Lemon is a good source of vitamin C, which can help improve blood vessel function.
Ginger has powerful anti-inflammatory properties that can help reduce pain and inflammation, as well as improve blood circulation.

Nutritional Information:

Calories: 95
Carbohydrates: 23g
Protein: 3g
Fat: 1g
Sugar: 12g
Sodium: 44mg

Tomato and Basil Juice

Ingredients:

3 medium tomatoes, chopped
1/2 cucumber
1/2 red bell pepper
1/4 cup fresh basil leaves

Instructions:

Wash all the ingredients thoroughly.
Chop the tomatoes, cucumber, and bell pepper into small pieces.
Put the ingredients into the juicer and extract the juice.
Pour the juice into a glass and enjoy!

Benefits:

Tomatoes are rich in lycopene, which can help reduce inflammation and improve heart health.
Cucumber is high in water and can help hydrate the body and reduce blood pressure.
Red bell pepper is high in vitamin C and can help improve blood vessel function.
Basil has anti-inflammatory properties and can help improve circulation.

Nutritional Information:

Calories: 86
Carbohydrates: 20g
Protein: 3g
Fat: 1g
Sugar: 12g
Sodium: 54mg

Beet and Carrot Juice

Ingredients:

1 medium beet, peeled and chopped
4 medium carrots, peeled and chopped
1/2 lemon, peeled
1-inch piece of fresh ginger, peeled

Instructions:

Wash all the ingredients thoroughly.
Chop the beet, carrots, and lemon into small pieces.
Put the ingredients into the juicer and extract the juice.
Pour the juice into a glass and enjoy!

Benefits:

Beets are rich in nitrates, which can help improve blood flow and lower
blood pressure.
Carrots are rich in antioxidants and can help reduce inflammation in the
body.
Lemon is a good source of vitamin C and can help improve heart health.
Ginger has anti-inflammatory properties and can help reduce the risk of
heart disease.

Nutritional Information:

Calories: 150
Carbohydrates: 37g
Protein: 3g
Fat: 1g
Sugar: 23g
Sodium: 129mg

Tomato, Basil, and Lemon Juice

Ingredients:

4 medium tomatoes
1/2 cup fresh basil leaves
1/2 lemon, peeled

Instructions:

Wash all the ingredients thoroughly.
Chop the tomatoes into small pieces.
Put the ingredients into the juicer and extract the juice.
Pour the juice into a glass and enjoy!

Benefits:

Tomatoes are high in lycopene, which can help lower cholesterol levels.
Basil is high in antioxidants and can help reduce inflammation in the body.

Nutritional Information:

Calories: 89
Carbohydrates: 21g
Protein: 4g
Fat: 1g
Sugar: 11g
Sodium: 21mg

Beet-Apple-Carrot Juice

Ingredients:

1 medium beets, peeled and chopped
1 medium apple, cored and chopped
2 medium carrots, peeled and chopped
1 inch ginger root, peeled
1/2 lemon, peeled

Instructions:

Wash all the ingredients thoroughly.
Chop the beets, apple, and carrots into small pieces.
Peel the ginger and lemon.
Put the ingredients into the juicer and extract the juice.
Pour the juice into a glass and enjoy!

Benefits:

Beetroot: contains nitrates that help to lower blood pressure and improve
circulation.
Apple: high in fiber, vitamin C, and antioxidants that support heart health.
Carrots: contain beta-carotene, vitamin A, and potassium that are
beneficial for heart health and circulation.
Ginger: has anti-inflammatory properties that can help to reduce
inflammation in the body.
Lemon: high in vitamin C that supports immune function and has
antioxidant properties that can protect against cell damage.

Nutritional Information:

Calories: 148
Protein: 3g
Fat: 1g
Carbohydrates: 36g
Sugar: 22g
Sodium: 140mg

Maintaining a healthy heart

Here are some tips for maintaining heart health through juicing and healthy lifestyle habits:

- **Focus on fruits and vegetables:** Juicing is an excellent way to incorporate more fruits and vegetables into your diet, which can help reduce the risk of heart disease. Choose fruits and vegetables that are high in fiber, antioxidants, and other heart-healthy nutrients, such as leafy greens, berries, and citrus fruits.
- **Increase your intake of heart-healthy fats:** Including foods like avocado, nuts, and seeds in your diet. These types of fats have been shown to lower inflammation and support cardiovascular health.
- **Avoid added sugars:** Many commercial juices contain added sugars, which can increase the risk of heart disease. Instead, make your juice at home using fresh, whole ingredients, and avoid adding any additional sweeteners.
- **Exercise regularly:** Exercise is essential for maintaining heart health. Aim to engage in at least 30 minutes of moderate-intensity physical activity on most days of the week. Some excellent choices for physical activity include walking, cycling, and swimming.
- To decrease the risk of heart disease, it is crucial to handle chronic stress effectively. Look for methods to manage stress, such as practicing meditation, deep breathing exercises, or yoga.
- Stopping smoking is a crucial measure in lowering the chance of developing heart disease. Smoking increases the risk of heart and blood vessel diseases, including coronary artery disease, heart attack, stroke, and peripheral artery disease. If you smoke, talk to your healthcare provider about strategies to quit.
- Restrict your intake of alcohol: Consuming excessive alcohol can raise blood pressure and contribute to the progression of heart disease. Limit your alcohol consumption to one or two drinks per day.

By incorporating these healthy habits into your routine, along with regular juicing using heart-healthy ingredients, you can help maintain and improve heart health, reducing the risk of developing heart disease and other cardiovascular conditions.

In conclusion, to maintain good overall health, it is important to prioritize heart health. The heart plays a vital role in the body, and when it is not functioning properly, it can cause a range of health issues including heart attacks, strokes, and heart failure. To reduce the risk of developing heart disease, it is important to make lifestyle changes such as eating a healthy diet, exercising regularly, and managing stress. Regular check-ups with a healthcare provider can also help identify risk factors and detect early signs of heart problems.

There are many reasons to prioritize heart health, including the fact that heart health is critical for overall health. Since the heart is responsible for pumping blood and oxygen throughout the body, it affects many different systems and organs. A healthy heart can reduce the risk of many health problems and improve overall well-being. Additionally, heart disease is preventable, and making lifestyle changes can significantly reduce the risk of developing heart disease.

Lifestyle changes can also help to improve heart health, even if you already have heart disease or are at risk of developing it. Exercise can strengthen the heart and lower blood pressure, while a heart-healthy diet can help to lower cholesterol levels. By making these changes, you can prevent or delay the progression of heart disease and improve outcomes.

Regular check-ups with a healthcare provider are also important for maintaining heart health. They can help identify risk factors for heart disease and detect early signs of heart problems, which can prevent or delay the progression of heart disease and improve outcomes.

Incorporating heart-healthy foods into your diet through juicing can be a convenient and delicious way to promote heart health. However, it is important to be mindful of portion sizes and calorie intake, as excessive calorie consumption can lead to weight gain and other health problems. Additionally, it is important to consult with a healthcare provider before making significant changes to your diet or starting a juicing regimen, particularly if you have a heart condition or are on medication. Foods that are high in antioxidants, such as blueberries, strawberries, spinach, and kale, can help protect the heart from damage. Other heart-healthy foods include beets, carrots, apples, and pomegranates, which are all high in nutrients that promote heart health.

Note: These recipes are not intended to treat or cure any medical condition. Please consult with your healthcare provider before making any significant changes to your diet.

Notes:

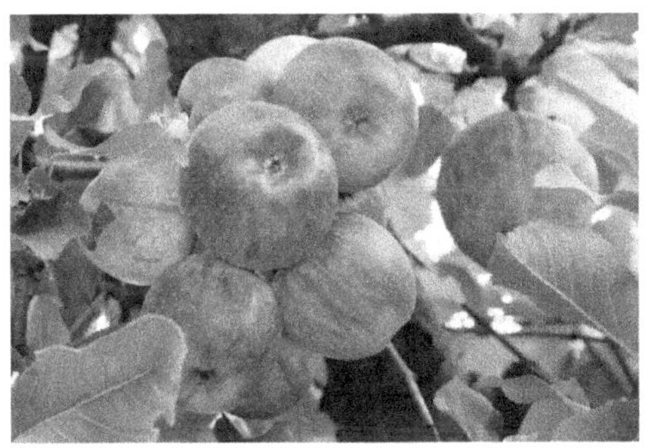

Improve Circulation

"The food you eat can either be the safest and most powerful form of medicine or the slowest form of poison." - Ann Wigmore

Circulation and your health

Circulation plays a crucial role in overall health and well-being. It is responsible for delivering oxygen and nutrients to all parts of the body, including the brain, muscles, and organs, and removing waste products and carbon dioxide.

Here are some reasons why circulation is essential for health and well-being:

- **Maintains organ function:** Adequate blood flow is essential for maintaining the function of vital organs such as the heart, brain, and kidneys. Poor circulation can lead to damage or dysfunction of these organs, increasing the risk of disease.

- **Promotes healing:** Blood flow is critical for healing and recovery from injuries, surgeries, and other health conditions. Proper circulation brings oxygen and nutrients to the site of injury or inflammation, promoting healing and reducing recovery time.

- **Supports brain function:** The brain is one of the most metabolically active organs in the body and requires a constant supply of oxygen and nutrients. Good circulation helps deliver these essential nutrients, supporting brain function and reducing the risk of cognitive decline.

- **Enhances immune function:** The immune system relies on blood flow to transport immune cells and antibodies to fight off infections and other threats to health. Good circulation helps support immune function and can reduce the risk of infection and disease.

- **Reduces the risk of cardiovascular disease:** Poor circulation can contribute to the development of cardiovascular disease, such as high blood pressure, heart attack, and stroke. By improving circulation, you can reduce the risk of these conditions and improve overall cardiovascular health.

By adopting healthy lifestyle habits, such as regular exercise, a healthy diet, and stress management techniques, you can help improve circulation and support overall health and well-being.

Do's:

- Incorporate plenty of fruits and vegetables that are high in antioxidants and anti-inflammatory compounds, such as berries, leafy greens, beets, and ginger.
- Consider adding citrus fruits like oranges and grapefruits, which contain high levels of vitamin C that can help strengthen blood vessels.
- Drink plenty of water to stay hydrated and support proper circulation.
- Consider adding spices like turmeric and cayenne pepper, which have been shown to improve circulation.

Don'ts:

- Avoid adding large amounts of high-sugar fruits like pineapples, mangoes, and bananas, high-sugar foods can contribute to inflammation and negatively impact blood sugar levels.
- Avoid adding excessive amounts of salt, salt can contribute to high blood pressure and negatively impact circulation.

Warnings:

- If you have any underlying health conditions, particularly related to the heart or circulation, it's important to speak with a healthcare professional before starting any new juicing regimen.
- Be aware that some medications, particularly blood thinners, can interact with certain fruits and vegetables, so it's important to speak with your healthcare provider about any potential risks.

Advice:

- Consider incorporating a variety of fruits and vegetables into your juices to ensure that you are getting a diverse range of nutrients that can support circulation.
- Aim to drink your juices immediately after juicing to minimize oxidation and ensure that you are getting the maximum nutritional benefit.
- Consider using a cold-pressed juicer, which can help preserve nutrients and enzymes that can be destroyed by heat or high-speed juicing.

Foods for your Circulation Juice

- **Beets:** Beets are rich in nitrates, which help to relax and widen blood vessels, resulting in lower blood pressure and improved blood flow.

- **Kale:** Kale is packed with antioxidants and anti-inflammatory compounds that help protect the heart from damage.

- **Spinach:** Spinach is a good source of magnesium; magnesium helps regulate blood pressure and maintain healthy heart function.

- **Carrots:** Carrots are high in beta-carotene; beta-carotene has been linked to a lower risk of heart disease.

- **Apples:** Apples are high in fiber and antioxidants; fiber and antioxidants have been shown to help reduce cholesterol levels and lower the risk of heart disease.

- **Blueberries:** Blueberries are packed with anthocyanins; anthocyanins have been shown to help reduce inflammation and improve circulation.

- **Pomegranates:** Pomegranates are rich in polyphenols; polyphenols have been shown to reduce the risk of heart disease by improving blood flow and reducing inflammation.

- **Tomatoes:** Tomatoes are rich in lycopene; lycopene has been linked to a reduced risk of heart disease.

- **Ginger:** Ginger has anti-inflammatory properties that can help reduce inflammation and improve heart health.

- **Garlic:** Garlic contains allicin, a compound that has been shown to lower cholesterol levels and reduce the risk of heart disease.

Boost your Circulation Juice

- **Beetroot Powder:** Beetroot is rich in nitrates, which can help improve blood flow and lower blood pressure. Adding beetroot powder to your juice can provide these benefits.

- **Cayenne Pepper Powder:** Cayenne pepper contains capsaicin, which can help improve blood circulation by widening blood vessels and increasing blood flow. However, use caution when adding cayenne pepper to your juice, as it can be quite spicy.

- **Ginger Powder:** Ginger has anti-inflammatory properties and can help improve circulation by promoting blood flow. It may also help reduce blood pressure and prevent blood clots.

- **Cinnamon Powder:** Cinnamon contains compounds that can help improve blood circulation by relaxing blood vessels and increasing blood flow. It may also help lower blood pressure and reduce inflammation.

- **Turmeric Powder:** Turmeric contains curcumin, which has anti-inflammatory properties and can help improve blood flow by promoting blood vessel health. It may also help reduce blood pressure and prevent blood clots.

Remember to always consult with a healthcare professional before adding any new supplements to your diet.

Red Juice

Ingredients:

2 beets
2 carrots
1/2 red bell pepper
1-inch piece of ginger

Instructions:

Wash all the ingredients thoroughly.
Peel the beetroots and carrots, and chop them into small pieces.
Remove the seeds from the red bell pepper, and cut it into small pieces.
Put the ingredients into the juicer and extract the juice.
Pour the juice into a glass and enjoy!

Benefits:

Beets are high in nitrates, which can help improve blood flow and circulation.
Carrots are rich in vitamin A and can help improve circulation.
Red bell pepper is a good source of vitamin C and can help improve blood flow.
Ginger has powerful anti-inflammatory properties that can help reduce pain and inflammation, as well as improve blood circulation.

Nutritional Information:

Calories: 130
Carbohydrates: 30g
Protein: 5g
Fat: 1g
Sugar: 16g
Sodium: 197mg

Beet and Carrot Juice

Ingredients:

2 medium beets, peeled and chopped
4 medium carrots, peeled and chopped
1/2 lemon, peeled
1-inch piece of ginger

Instructions:

Wash all the ingredients thoroughly.
Chop the beets and carrots into small pieces.
Put the ingredients into the juicer and extract the juice.
Pour the juice into a glass and enjoy!

Benefits:

Beets are high in nitrates, which can help improve blood flow and lower blood pressure.
Carrots are rich in beta-carotene, which can help improve circulation.
Lemon is a good source of vitamin C and can help improve blood vessel function.
Ginger has powerful anti-inflammatory properties that can help reduce pain and inflammation, as well as improve blood circulation.

Nutritional Information:

Calories: 178
Carbohydrates: 43g
Protein: 5g
Fat: 1g
Sugar: 25g
Sodium: 251mg

Orange and Beetroot Juice

Ingredients:

2 medium oranges, peeled and chopped
2 medium beets, peeled and chopped
1/2 lemon, peeled
1-inch piece of ginger

Instructions:

Wash all the ingredients thoroughly.
Chop the oranges and beets into small pieces.
Put the ingredients into the juicer and extract the juice.
Pour the juice into a glass and enjoy!

Benefits:

Oranges are high in vitamin C, which can help improve blood vessel function and reduce inflammation.
Beets are high in nitrates, which can help improve blood flow and lower blood pressure.
Lemon is a good source of vitamin C and can help improve blood vessel function.
Ginger has powerful anti-inflammatory properties that can help reduce pain and inflammation, as well as improve blood circulation.

Nutritional Information:

Calories: 181
Carbohydrates: 44g
Protein: 5g
Fat: 1g
Sugar: 27g
Sodium: 229mg

Beet and Berry Juice

Ingredients:

1 medium beet, peeled and chopped
1 cup mixed berries (blueberries, raspberries, blackberries)
1-inch piece of fresh ginger, peeled

Instructions:

Wash all the ingredients thoroughly.
Chop the beet into small pieces.
Put the ingredients into the juicer and extract the juice.
Pour the juice into a glass and enjoy!

Benefits:

Beets are rich in nitrates, which can help improve blood flow and circulation.
Berries are rich in antioxidants, which may aid in reducing inflammation within the body.
Ginger has powerful anti-inflammatory properties that can help reduce pain and inflammation, as well as improve blood circulation.

Nutritional Information:

Calories: 135
Carbohydrates: 33g
Protein: 2g
Fat: 1g
Sugar: 19g
Sodium: 59mg

Citrus Juice with Orange and Grapefruit

Ingredients:

2 medium oranges, peeled
1 large grapefruit, peeled
1-inch piece of fresh ginger, peeled

Instructions:

Wash all the ingredients thoroughly.
Chop the oranges and grapefruit into small pieces.
Put the ingredients into the juicer and extract the juice.
Pour the juice into a glass and enjoy!

Benefits:

Oranges are high in vitamin C, which can help improve blood flow and
circulation.
Grapefruit is low in calories and can help lower blood pressure.
Ginger has powerful anti-inflammatory properties that can help reduce pain
and inflammation, as well as improve blood circulation.

Nutritional Information:

Calories: 141
Carbohydrates: 34g
Protein: 2g
Fat: 1g
Sugar: 22g
Sodium: 0mg

How can I improve my circulation?

Here are some tips for promoting circulation through juicing and healthy lifestyle habits:

- **Incorporate fruits and vegetables with circulation-boosting nutrients:** Certain nutrients, such as vitamin C, vitamin E, and flavonoids, have been shown to improve circulation. Incorporate fruits and vegetables that are high in these nutrients into your juices, such as citrus fruits, berries, leafy greens, and beets.

- **Add spices and herbs:** Certain spices and herbs, such as cayenne pepper, ginger, and garlic, have been shown to improve circulation by increasing blood flow and reducing inflammation. Add these ingredients to your juices for an extra circulation boost.

- **Stay hydrated:** Adequate hydration is essential for maintaining healthy blood flow. Drink plenty of water throughout the day to support circulation.

- **Exercise regularly:** Exercise is one of the most effective ways to improve circulation. Aim for at least 30 minutes of moderate-intensity exercise most days of the week, such as walking, cycling, or swimming.

- **Quitting smoking:** Smoking can cause harm to blood vessels and reduce blood flow, leading to an increased risk of circulatory issues. If you smoke, it is advisable to speak with your healthcare provider to explore ways to quit.

- **Manage your stress:** Effective stress management is crucial for promoting good blood flow and circulation, as chronic stress can lead to the constriction of blood vessels. Incorporating stress-reducing practices like meditation, deep breathing exercises, or yoga can help you manage stress and support healthy circulation.

By incorporating these healthy habits into your routine, along with regular juicing using circulation-boosting ingredients, you can help promote healthy blood flow and support overall health and well-being.

In conclusion, improving circulation is vital for overall health and well-being. Adequate blood flow delivers essential nutrients and oxygen to all parts of the body while removing waste products, promoting healing, supporting brain function, enhancing immune function, and reducing the risk of cardiovascular disease.

By adopting healthy lifestyle habits, such as a regular exercise routine, a balanced diet rich in fruits and vegetables, and stress management techniques, you can help improve circulation and support your overall health.

When it comes to creating a circulation-boosting juice, incorporating a variety of fruits and vegetables is essential to ensure that you're getting a diverse range of nutrients that can support circulation. Beets, kale, spinach, carrots, apples, blueberries, pomegranates, tomatoes, ginger, and garlic are all great choices for a circulation-boosting juice.

Adding beetroot powder, cayenne pepper powder, ginger powder, cinnamon powder, or turmeric powder to your juice can provide additional benefits for improving blood flow and lowering blood pressure. However, it's crucial to consult with a healthcare professional before adding any new supplements, especially if you have an underlying health condition.

It's important to remember to avoid excessive amounts of high-sugar fruits and salt, which can negatively impact circulation. If you have an underlying health condition related to the heart or circulation, it's crucial to speak with a healthcare professional before starting any new juicing regimen.

By following these do's and don'ts and incorporating circulation-boosting foods and supplements, you can create a delicious and nutritious juice that supports your overall health and well-being.

Note: These recipes are not intended to treat or cure any medical condition. Please consult with your healthcare provider before making any significant changes to your diet.

Notes:_______________________

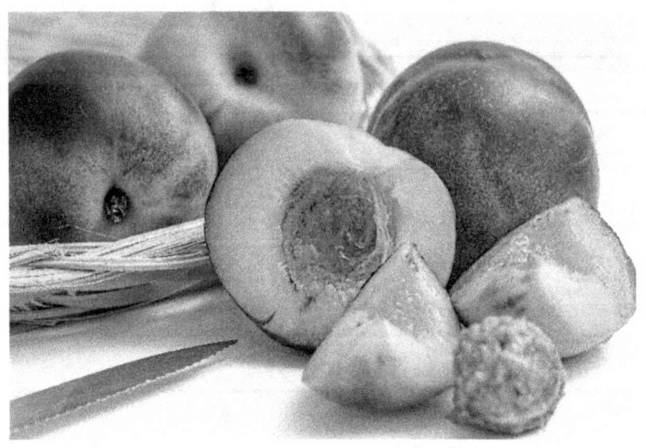

Strong Bones

"Good nutrition is essential for the development and maintenance of healthy bones throughout the life cycle." - National Osteoporosis Foundation. (2017).

Understanding Bone Health

As we age, our bones naturally begin to lose density and strength. This can lead to an increased risk of fractures and osteoporosis, a condition where bones become weak and brittle. Bone loss typically begins in our mid-30s and can accelerate as we get older, particularly in postmenopausal women.

Maintaining good bone health is important for several reasons. First, strong bones can help prevent fractures and injuries, which can lead to a loss of independence and mobility in older adults. This is especially important as we age, as falls are a common cause of injury among older adults and can have serious consequences. Second, good bone health is essential for maintaining overall physical activity and quality of life. Strong bones allow us to participate in activities we enjoy, like walking, hiking, and dancing, and can help us maintain our independence as we age. Finally, strong bones can help prevent osteoporosis and other age-related bone diseases. Osteoporosis is a common condition in older adults, particularly women, and can lead to fractures, chronic pain, and disability.

There are several things you can do to maintain good bone health as you age. These include:

- **Getting enough calcium and vitamin D:** Calcium and vitamin D are essential for building and maintaining strong bones. Calcium is the most important mineral for bone health, and the body needs vitamin D to absorb and use it effectively. Foods such as dairy products, leafy greens, and fortified cereals are good sources of calcium, while vitamin D can be found in fatty fish, egg yolks, and fortified foods. Supplements may be necessary to achieve adequate levels of these nutrients, particularly for older adults who may have trouble getting enough vitamin D through their diet or sunlight exposure.

- **Exercising regularly:** Weight-bearing exercises, such as walking, jogging, and strength training, can help improve bone density and strength. Exercise can also help improve balance and coordination, which can reduce the risk of falls and fractures.

- **Quitting smoking:** Smoking has been linked to a higher risk of osteoporosis and bone fractures. Quitting smoking is one of the best things you can do for your bone health, as well as for your overall health.

- **Limiting alcohol consumption:** Drinking too much alcohol can decrease bone density and increase the risk of fractures. Women should limit alcohol intake to one drink per day, while men should limit intake to two drinks per day.

- **Getting regular bone density screenings:** Bone density screenings can help detect osteoporosis and other bone diseases early, when they are most treatable. Talk to your healthcare provider about when to start getting screened and how often to repeat the test.

Juicing can provide a wide range of nutrients that are beneficial for bone health. Here are some key nutrients that are important for maintaining healthy bones:

- **Calcium:** This mineral is essential for building and maintaining strong bones. Calcium is found in many foods, including dairy products, leafy greens, and some types of fish. Adding calcium-rich ingredients like kale, collard greens, broccoli, and almond milk to your juices can help boost your calcium intake.

- **Vitamin D:** This vitamin is essential for the absorption of calcium in the body. Vitamin D is primarily obtained from sunlight, but it can also be found in fatty fish, eggs, and fortified foods. Adding ingredients like mushrooms, fortified orange juice, and salmon to your juices can help increase your vitamin D intake.

- **Vitamin K:** This vitamin is important for bone health because it helps regulate calcium absorption and utilization in the body. Vitamin K is found in leafy greens like spinach, kale, and Swiss chard, and can be added to your juices for an extra boost.

- **Magnesium:** This mineral is important for bone health because it helps regulate calcium absorption and utilization in the body.

Do's:

- Choose calcium-rich vegetables such as kale, collard greens, broccoli, and bok choy for your juice.
- Include vitamin D-rich vegetables such as spinach, mushrooms, and kale in your juice.
- Add magnesium-rich ingredients like almonds, spinach, and avocado to your juice.
- Drink plenty of water alongside your juice to stay hydrated and support healthy bones.
- Combine your juice with other healthy foods, and exercise regularly for optimal bone health.

Don'ts:

- Avoid adding too much sugar to your juice, as it can interfere with calcium absorption and lead to bone loss.
- Do not rely solely on juice as your main source of nutrients for bone health.
- Avoid using vegetables that are high in oxalates, such as spinach and Swiss chard, which can bind to calcium and prevent the absorption of calcium.
- Do not add too much salt to your juice, as excessive sodium intake can lead to bone loss.

Warnings and advise:

- Consult with your doctor before starting any juicing regimen, especially if you have a history of osteoporosis or other bone conditions.
- Juicing may not be appropriate for individuals with certain medical conditions, such as kidney disease or diabetes.
- Drinking large amounts of certain juices, such as beet juice, may cause temporary discoloration of urine and stools.
- Use a variety of fruits and vegetables in your juice to ensure you are getting a range of nutrients that support bone health.
- Consider adding a source of protein to your juice, such as Greek yogurt or protein powder, to further support bone health.
- Store your juice properly to maintain its nutrient content and prevent bacterial growth.
- Drink your juice soon after making it to maximize its nutrient content.

Foods for Bone Health

- **Spinach** - Spinach is rich in vitamin K, vitamin K essential for bone health. Vitamin K helps in building strong bones by increasing calcium absorption and reducing the loss of calcium through urine.

- **Kale** - Kale is another excellent source of vitamin K. It also contains calcium, magnesium, and vitamin C, all of which are crucial for bone health.

- **Broccoli** - Broccoli is rich in vitamin C, vitamin C is essential to produce collagen, a protein that provides strength and flexibility to bones.

- **Carrots** - Carrots are a good source of vitamin A, vitamin A is necessary for bone growth and development. Vitamin A also helps in maintaining healthy skin and eyesight.

- **Sweet Potatoes** - Sweet potatoes are a rich source of vitamin A and potassium, vitamin A and potassium are essential for bone health.

- **Beets** - Beets are high in potassium and magnesium, both of which are essential for strong bones. They also contain iron, iron is essential to the production of hemoglobin in the blood.

- **Ginger** - Ginger is rich in antioxidants, antioxidants can help reduce inflammation and improve bone health. Ginger also contains magnesium, potassium, and vitamin B6.

- **Turmeric** - Turmeric is rich in curcumin, curcumin has anti-inflammatory properties. It can help reduce inflammation in the joints and improve bone health.

- **Cabbage** - Cabbage is a good source of vitamin K, vitamin K is essential for bone health. It also contains calcium and magnesium, both of which are essential for strong bones.

- **Pineapple** - Pineapple contains bromelain, an enzyme that helps in breaking down proteins. This can help reduce inflammation and improve bone health. Pineapple is also a good source of vitamin C, vitamin C is essential for collagen production.

Boost your Bone Health Juice

- **Collagen powder:** Collagen is a protein that helps to maintain bone strength and joint health.

- **Calcium powder:** Calcium is an essential mineral that is important for building and maintaining strong bones.

- **Vitamin D powder:** Vitamin D helps the body absorb calcium and is important for maintaining bone health.

- **Magnesium powder:** Magnesium is an essential mineral that helps to support bone health and can help prevent bone loss.

- **Vitamin K2 powder:** Vitamin K2 helps to regulate calcium in the body and can help to support bone health.

- **Turmeric powder:** Turmeric has anti-inflammatory properties that can help to reduce inflammation and support bone health.

- **Ginger powder:** Ginger has anti-inflammatory properties that can help to reduce inflammation and support bone health.

- **Cinnamon powder:** Cinnamon has anti-inflammatory properties that can help to reduce inflammation and support bone health.

- **Maca powder:** Maca is a root vegetable that is high in vitamins and minerals and can help to support bone health.

- **Green tea powder:** Green tea is high in antioxidants and has anti-inflammatory properties that can help to support bone health.

Remember to always consult with a healthcare professional before adding any new supplements to your diet.

Green Bone Juice

Ingredients:

1 cup kale
1 cup spinach
1 medium cucumber
1 medium green apple
1/2 lemon, peeled
1 inch piece of ginger
1 tablespoon chia seeds

Instructions:

Wash all the ingredients thoroughly.
Chop the kale, spinach, cucumber, and green apple into small pieces.
Put all the ingredients, except chia seeds, into the juicer and extract the juice.
Stir in the chia seeds.
Pour the juice into a glass and enjoy!

Benefits:

Kale and spinach are high in calcium, vitamin K, and other minerals that are essential for bone health.
Cucumbers are a good source of silica, which is important for maintaining strong bones and healthy connective tissues.
Green apples are high in antioxidants, which can help reduce inflammation and protect bone cells from damage.
Lemons and ginger have anti-inflammatory properties that can help reduce pain and stiffness in the joints.
Chia seeds are high in omega-3 fatty acids and minerals like calcium and magnesium, which are important for bone health.

Nutritional Information:

Calories: 170
Carbohydrates: 36g
Protein: 6g
Fat: 3g
Sugar: 20g
Sodium: 60mg

Berry Bone Juice

Ingredients:

1 cup strawberries
1/2 cup blueberries
1/2 cup raspberries
1 medium carrot
1 medium orange
1 inch piece of turmeric
1 tablespoon flaxseed

Instructions:

Wash all the ingredients thoroughly.
Chop the strawberries, carrot, and orange into small pieces.
Put all the ingredients, except flaxseed, into the juicer and extract the juice.
Stir in the flaxseed.
Pour the juice into a glass and enjoy!

Benefits:

Strawberries, blueberries, and raspberries are rich in vitamin C, which is essential for collagen formation in bones and connective tissues.
Carrots are a good source of vitamin A, which helps in the absorption of calcium and other minerals.
Oranges are high in vitamin C and flavonoids, which can help reduce inflammation and improve bone density.
Turmeric has anti-inflammatory and antioxidant properties that can help reduce pain and inflammation in the joints.
Flaxseed is rich in omega-3 fatty acids, lignans, and fiber, which can help reduce bone loss and improve bone density.

Nutritional Information:

Calories: 170
Carbohydrates: 36g
Protein: 3g
Fat: 3g
Sugar: 20g
Sodium: 50mg

Bone Juice

Ingredients:

2 cups kale
1 large carrot
1/2 cucumber
1/2 apple
1/2-inch ginger root
1/2 lemon
1/2 cup broccoli

Instructions:

Wash all the ingredients thoroughly.
Chop everything into small pieces.
Put all the ingredients into the juicer and extract the juice.
Stir the juice well and pour it into a glass.

Benefits:

Kale is a great source of calcium, vitamin K, and other minerals.
Carrots are high in vitamin A and potassium, which can help improve bone density and strength.
Cucumbers are a good source of silica, which is important for maintaining strong bones and healthy connective tissues.
Apples are high in antioxidants, which can help reduce inflammation and protect bone cells from damage.
Ginger root has anti-inflammatory properties that can help reduce pain and stiffness in the joints.
Lemons are a good source of vitamin C, which can help boost the immune system and support bone health.
Broccoli is high in calcium, magnesium, and other minerals that are essential for bone health.

Nutritional Information:

Calories: 118
Carbohydrates: 28g
Protein: 5g
Fat: 1g
Sugar: 14g
Sodium: 71mg

Phosphorus Punch Juice:

Ingredients:

2 cups bok choy
1 large carrot
1/2 cup grapes
1/2-inch ginger root
1/2 lemon

Instructions:

Wash all the ingredients thoroughly.
Cut the bok choy into small pieces.
Cut the carrot and ginger into small pieces.
Juice the bok choy, carrot, ginger, grapes, and lemon in a juicer.
Stir the juice well and serve immediately.

Benefits:

Bok choy is a great source of phosphorus, a mineral that is essential for strong bones and teeth.
Carrots are high in vitamin A, which helps the body absorb calcium and promote bone growth.
Grapes contain resveratrol, an antioxidant that has been shown to increase bone density and prevent bone loss.
Ginger has anti-inflammatory properties that can help reduce joint pain and stiffness.
Lemon is high in vitamin C, which is important for collagen production and bone health.

Nutritional Information:

Calories: 140
Carbohydrates: 33g
Protein: 3g
Fat: 1g
Sugar: 19g
Sodium: 95mg

Vitamin D Booster Juice:

Ingredients:

2 cups collard greens
1 large beetroot
1/2 cup strawberries
1/2-inch turmeric root
1/2 lemon

Instructions:

Wash all the ingredients thoroughly.
Chop the collard greens, beetroot, and turmeric root into small pieces.
Put all the ingredients into the juicer and extract the juice.
Pour the juice into a glass and enjoy!
Benefits:

Collard greens are a good source of vitamin D, which helps the body absorb calcium and maintain strong bones.
Beetroot is high in potassium and magnesium, which are important minerals for bone health.
Strawberries are rich in vitamin C, which is essential for collagen production and bone strength.
Turmeric root has anti-inflammatory properties that can help reduce pain and inflammation in the joints.
Lemon is high in vitamin C and can help improve the absorption of nutrients in the body.

Nutritional Information:

Calories: 150
Carbohydrates: 35g
Protein: 5g
Fat: 1g
Sugar: 20g
Sodium: 80mg

In conclusion, maintaining good bone health is crucial for overall health and well-being, especially as we age. The importance of maintaining good bone health cannot be overstated, as strong bones help prevent fractures, maintain independence, and prevent bone diseases like osteoporosis.

As we grow older, the density and strength of our bones naturally decrease, making it more important than ever to prioritize our bone health. Thankfully, there are several effective ways to maintain good bone health, including getting enough calcium and vitamin D, engaging in regular exercise, and limiting alcohol consumption.

Juicing can also play a significant role in promoting good bone health by providing key nutrients like calcium, vitamin D, vitamin K, and magnesium, all of which are essential for maintaining strong bones. When juicing for bone health, it is important to choose calcium-rich vegetables, include vitamin D-rich ingredients, and avoid adding too much sugar or salt.

Before starting any juicing regimen, it is crucial to consult with your healthcare provider, particularly if you have a history of bone conditions. Incorporating bone-healthy foods like spinach, kale, and salmon into your diet can also help support good bone health.

By following these tips and taking proactive steps to maintain strong bones, you can reduce your risk of bone-related health problems and enjoy a better quality of life as you age. Remember, maintaining good bone health is an ongoing process that requires consistent effort and dedication, but the benefits are well worth it in the long run.

Note: These recipes are not intended to treat or cure any medical condition. Please consult with your healthcare provider before making any significant changes to your diet.

Notes:_______________________

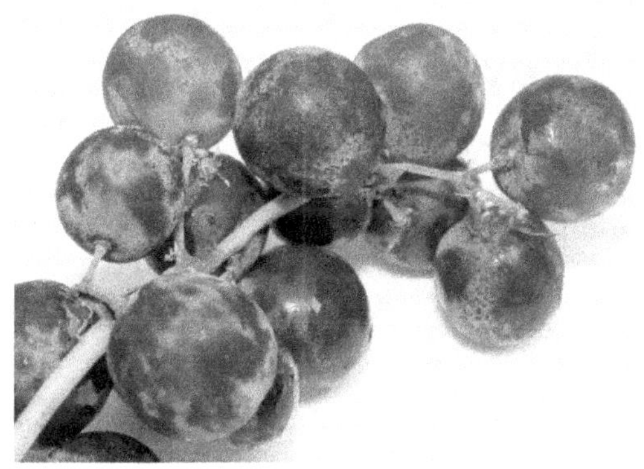

Cleanse Your System

"Juice fasting is the fastest way to restore the body and mind to health." - Paavo Airola

What is detoxifying or cleansing?

Detoxification refers to the process of removing toxins and other harmful substances from the body. Juicing can be an effective way to support the body's natural detoxification processes and promote overall health and well-being. Here are some benefits of detoxifying your body through juicing:

- **Supports liver function:** The liver is responsible for filtering toxins and waste products from the blood. Juicing can provide the liver with essential nutrients and antioxidants, supporting its ability to detoxify the body.

- **Boosts energy levels:** When toxins build up in the body, it can lead to fatigue and low energy levels. By removing these harmful substances through juicing, you can help boost energy levels and improve overall vitality.

- **Improves digestion:** Juicing can help promote healthy digestion by providing the body with essential nutrients and enzymes that support the digestive process. It can also help remove toxins and waste products from the digestive tract, reducing the risk of constipation and other digestive problems.

- **Reduces inflammation:** Toxins in the body can lead to inflammation, which can contribute to a wide range of health problems. Juicing can provide the body with anti-inflammatory compounds, such as ginger and turmeric, helping to reduce inflammation and promote overall health.

- **Supports immune function:** When toxins build up in the body, it can weaken the immune system and increase the risk of infection and disease. Juicing can provide the body with essential vitamins and minerals that support immune function and help reduce the risk of illness.

By incorporating juicing into your daily routine, you can help support the body's natural detoxification processes and promote overall health and well-being. It is essential to also adopt healthy lifestyle habits, such as a balanced diet, regular exercise, and stress management, to support optimal health.

Do's:

- Choose fresh, organic fruits and vegetables for juicing.
- Incorporate a variety of colors and types of produce to ensure you get a wide range of nutrients.
- Drink plenty of water alongside your juices to stay hydrated.
- Consult with a healthcare professional before starting any cleanse or detox program.
- Ease into and out of a juice cleanse with lighter meals, like salads and steamed vegetables.

Don'ts:

- Avoid juicing fruits that are high in sugar, as they can cause blood sugar spikes and lead to energy crashes. Stick to low-sugar fruits like berries and apples.
- Don't rely solely on juice for long periods of time, as it can lead to nutrient deficiencies and other health issues.
- Avoid juicing cruciferous vegetables like broccoli, cauliflower, and cabbage in large amounts, as they can cause gas and bloating.

Warnings and Advice:

- If you have any health conditions or are taking medication, consult with a healthcare professional before starting any cleanse or detox program.
- Don't consume unpasteurized juices or juice from sources that are not reputable, as they can contain harmful bacteria.
- Be mindful of your body's response to a cleanse or detox program. If you experience any negative symptoms, like headaches or digestive issues, stop the program and consult with a healthcare professional.
- While juicing can be a healthy addition to your diet, it is not a magic solution for weight loss or detoxification. A balanced diet with whole foods is important for long-term health.

Foods for your Cleanse Juice

- **Lemon:** High in vitamin C and antioxidants, lemon juice can help detoxify the liver and aid digestion.

- **Ginger:** Contains anti-inflammatory compounds that can help reduce inflammation in the body and improve circulation.

- **Carrots:** Rich in vitamin A, carrots can help support liver function and promote healthy skin.

- **Kale:** Loaded with antioxidants, kale can help reduce oxidative stress and support liver health.

- **Beets:** High in nitrates, beets can help improve blood flow and support detoxification.

- **Cucumbers:** High in water and fiber, cucumbers can help flush out toxins and support healthy digestion.

- **Apples:** High in soluble fiber and antioxidants, apples can help regulate blood sugar levels and support liver function.

- **Parsley:** Rich in chlorophyll, parsley can help detoxify the body and support kidney function.

- **Pineapple:** Contains digestive enzymes that can help improve digestion and reduce inflammation.

- **Spinach:** High in antioxidants and nutrients, spinach can help protect against cellular damage and support liver function.

Boost your Cleanse Juice

- **Wheatgrass powder:** Wheatgrass is a popular ingredient in detox and cleansing diets. It is high in chlorophyll, which has been shown to have cleansing and detoxifying effects on the body.

- **Spirulina powder:** Spirulina is a type of blue-green algae that is rich in antioxidants and anti-inflammatory compounds. It has been shown to have detoxifying effects on the body and can help support liver function.

- **Chlorella powder:** Chlorella is another type of green algae that is high in chlorophyll and antioxidants. It has been shown to help support liver function and promote detoxification.

- **Psyllium husk powder:** Psyllium husk is a type of soluble fiber that is commonly used to support digestive health and promote regularity. It can also help to remove toxins from the body.

- **Dandelion root powder:** Dandelion root has long been used in traditional medicine for its diuretic properties, which can help to flush toxins from the body. It is also rich in antioxidants and can help to support liver function.

It is important to note that while these powders can be beneficial for cleansing, they should be used in moderation and under the guidance of a healthcare professional. It's also important to maintain a balanced and healthy diet while doing any kind of cleansing or detox program.

Cleansing Juice

Ingredients:

2 cucumbers
2 green apples
1/2 lemon, peeled
1/2 inch piece of turmeric

Instructions:

Wash all the ingredients thoroughly.
Chop the cucumbers and green apples into small pieces.
Peel the lemon and turmeric and cut it into small pieces.
Put the ingredients into the juicer and extract the juice.
Pour the juice into a glass and enjoy!

Benefits:

Cucumbers are rich in water and can help flush out toxins from the body.
Green apples are low in sugar and can help improve digestion.
Lemon is a good source of vitamin C and can help detoxify the liver.
Turmeric has anti-inflammatory properties and can help improve liver
function.

Nutritional Information:

Calories: 167
Carbohydrates: 43g
Protein: 2g
Fat: 1g
Sugar: 30g
Sodium: 8mg

Green Vegetable Juice

Ingredients:

1 cucumber
2 celery stalks
1/2 green apple
1/2 lemon, peeled
1 cup kale
1 cup spinach

Instructions:

Wash all the ingredients thoroughly.
The cucumber and celery should be sliced into small pieces.
Remove the core and seeds of the apple, and cut it into small pieces.
Put the ingredients into the juicer and extract the juice.
Pour the juice into a glass and enjoy!

Benefits:

Cucumber and celery are high in water and can help hydrate the body and flush out toxins.
Green apple is low in sugar and can help improve digestion.
Lemon is a good source of vitamin C and can help improve liver function.
Kale and spinach are rich in chlorophyll and can help detoxify the body.

Nutritional Information:

Calories: 89
Carbohydrates: 20g
Protein: 3g
Fat: 1g
Sugar: 10g
Sodium: 131mg

Pineapple and Mint Juice

Ingredients:

2 cups pineapple chunks
1/2 cucumber
1/4 cup fresh mint leaves
1/2 lemon, peeled

Instructions:

Wash all the ingredients thoroughly.
Chop the cucumber into small pieces.
Put the ingredients into the juicer and extract the juice.
Pour the juice into a glass and enjoy!

Benefits:

Pineapple is rich in enzymes that can help improve digestion and detoxify the body.
Cucumber is high in water and can help hydrate the body and flush out toxins.
Mint has a refreshing flavor and can help improve digestion.
Lemon is a good source of vitamin C and can help improve liver function.

Nutritional Information:

Calories: 128
Carbohydrates: 32g
Protein: 2g
Fat: 1g
Sugar: 22g
Sodium: 7mg

Apple and Cucumber Juice

Ingredients:

2 medium green apples, cored and chopped
1/2 cucumber
1/2 lemon, peeled
1/4 cup fresh mint leaves

Instructions:

Wash all the ingredients thoroughly.
Chop the apples and cucumber into small pieces.
Put the ingredients into the juicer and extract the juice.
Pour the juice into a glass and enjoy!

Benefits:

Apples are rich in fiber and can help improve digestion and cleanse the liver.
Cucumber is an excellent detoxifier, due to its high-water content and the presence of digestive enzymes. It helps to flush out toxins from the body and promote good digestion.
Lemon is a good source of vitamin C and can help improve liver function.
Mint has anti-inflammatory properties and can help soothe the digestive system.

Nutritional Information:

Calories: 127
Carbohydrates: 32g
Protein: 2g
Fat: 1g
Sugar: 22g
Sodium: 33mg

Green Juice with Kale and Celery

Ingredients:

2 cups kale
2 celery stalks
1 green apple, cored and chopped
1/2 lemon, peeled
1-inch piece of fresh ginger, peeled

Instructions:

Wash all the ingredients thoroughly.
The celery and apple should be chopped into small pieces.
Put the ingredients into the juicer and extract the juice.
Pour the juice into a glass and enjoy!

Benefits:

Kale is a great source of vitamins and antioxidants, which can help cleanse the body.
Celery is high in water and can help flush out toxins from the body.
Green apples are rich in fiber and can help improve digestion.

Nutritional Information:

Calories: 103
Carbohydrates: 26g
Protein: 3g
Fat: 1g
Sugar: 16g
Sodium: 105mg

Beet, Pineapple, and Ginger Juice

Ingredients:

1 medium beet, peeled and chopped
1 cup fresh pineapple chunks
1-inch piece of fresh ginger, peeled and chopped

Instructions:

Wash and prepare all ingredients.
Run the beet, pineapple, and ginger through a juicer.
Stir the juice well.
Serve over ice, if desired.

Benefits:

Beet: Beets are a root vegetable that are high in vitamins and minerals, including folate, iron, and potassium. They are also known for their ability to support liver function and reduce inflammation.
Pineapple: Pineapple is a tropical fruit that is high in vitamin C, manganese, and bromelain, an enzyme that can aid in digestion and reduce inflammation.
Ginger: Ginger is a root that has anti-inflammatory and antioxidant properties. It is commonly used in traditional medicine to aid digestion and reduce nausea.

Calories: 83
Carbohydrates: 20 g
Total Fat: 0.5 g
Fat: 0.5 g
Sugars: 15 g
Sodium: 63 mg

Why cleansing is important

Incorporating cleansing juices into your daily routine can help support the body's natural detoxification processes and promote overall health and well-being. Here are some tips for incorporating cleansing juices into your daily routine:

- **Start with simple recipes:** If you are new to juicing, start with simple recipes that use a few ingredients. This will make it easier to get started and help you develop a taste for fresh juices.

- **Choose nutrient-dense ingredients:** When making cleansing juices, choose nutrient-dense ingredients that are rich in vitamins, minerals, and antioxidants. Some examples include leafy greens, beets, carrots, and citrus fruits.

- **Make it a habit:** To get the most benefits from cleansing juices, make it a daily habit. Try incorporating a juice into your morning routine or as an afternoon snack.

- **Prepare ahead of time:** To save time, prepare your ingredients ahead of time. Wash and chop your fruits and vegetables, so they are ready to go when you are.

- **Experiment with different flavors:** Juicing is a fun and creative process, so don't be afraid to experiment with different flavors and combinations. Mix and match different fruits and vegetables until you find the flavors you enjoy.

- **Listen to your body:** As you start incorporating cleansing juices into your daily routine, pay attention to how your body feels. If you experience any adverse reactions or discomfort, reduce the amount or frequency of your juices, or speak with a healthcare provider.

By incorporating these tips into your routine, you can help make juicing a part of your daily routine and support your body's natural detoxification processes.

In conclusion, detoxifying or cleansing the body can have numerous benefits for overall health and well-being. Juicing is an effective way to support the body's natural detoxification processes and provide it with essential nutrients and antioxidants. By incorporating a variety of fresh, organic fruits and vegetables into your daily routine, you can help support liver function, boost energy levels, improve digestion, reduce inflammation, and support immune function.

However, it's important to be mindful of your body's response to a cleanse or detox program and to consult with a healthcare professional before starting any new regimen, especially if you have underlying health conditions or are taking medication. Additionally, it's crucial not to rely solely on juice for long periods of time, as it can lead to nutrient deficiencies and other health issues. A balanced diet with whole foods is essential for long-term health.

When it comes to juicing, it's important to choose low-sugar fruits and vegetables, incorporate a variety of colors and types of produce, and drink plenty of water alongside your juices to stay hydrated. Be mindful of foods to include and avoid in your juices and consider boosting their cleansing power with superfood powders like wheatgrass, spirulina, chlorella, psyllium husk, and dandelion root.

Overall, while juicing can be a healthy addition to your diet, it's not a magic solution for weight loss or detoxification. It's essential to adopt healthy lifestyle habits, such as a balanced diet, regular exercise, and stress management, to support optimal health. By making these changes, you can help support your body's natural detoxification processes and promote overall health and well-being.

Note: These recipes are not intended to treat or cure any medical condition. Please consult with your healthcare provider before making any significant changes to your diet.

Notes:

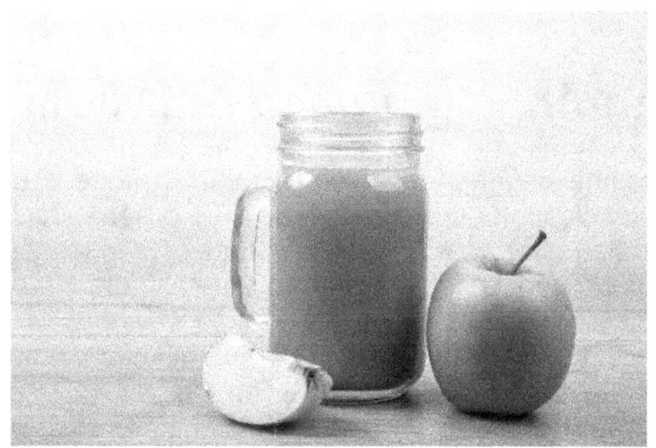

Youthful Nutrition

*"Those who do not find time for exercise will have to find time for illness." -
Edward Smith-Stanley*

Understanding aging and nutrition

All living organisms experience aging, a natural process of deterioration and degeneration. Aging is characterized by the gradual decline in physical and mental function over time. The aging process is influenced by a variety of factors, including genetics, lifestyle, and environmental factors.

One of the main factors that contribute to aging is oxidative stress. This occurs when there is an imbalance between free radicals (molecules with unpaired electrons) and antioxidants (molecules that neutralize free radicals) in the body. When there are too many free radicals and not enough antioxidants, it can lead to damage to cells and tissues, which can contribute to aging.

Another factor that contributes to aging is inflammation. Chronic inflammation can lead to damage to cells and tissues and has been linked to a variety of age-related diseases, including heart disease, cancer, and Alzheimer's disease.

There are several lifestyle habits that can help slow down the aging process. These include:

1. Eating a healthy diet that is rich in fruits and vegetables, whole grains, and lean proteins.
2. Exercising regularly to maintain physical fitness and mobility.
3. Managing stress through relaxation techniques such as meditation, yoga, or deep breathing exercises.
4. Getting enough sleep to allow the body to repair and regenerate.
5. Avoiding harmful habits such as smoking and excessive alcohol consumption.
6. Using sunscreen to protect the skin from damage caused by UV radiation.
7. Taking steps to reduce exposure to environmental toxins, such as air pollution and chemicals in household products.

Juicing can also be a beneficial way to slow down the aging process, as it provides a concentrated source of antioxidants and other nutrients that can help reduce oxidative stress and inflammation in the body. Incorporating antioxidant-rich fruits and vegetables such as blueberries, kale, spinach, and carrots into your juicing regimen can be especially beneficial for slowing down the aging process.

Do's:

- Incorporate a variety of colorful fruits and vegetables in your juices, as they are high in antioxidants that can help fight free radicals and slow down the aging process.
- Consider adding anti-aging superfoods such as goji berries, acai berries, chia seeds, and turmeric to your juices.
- Choose organic produce to reduce exposure to harmful pesticides and chemicals.
- Hydrate with plenty of water, in addition to your juices, to support healthy skin and overall health.
- Consider incorporating low-sugar green juices into your routine, as excess sugar consumption can contribute to premature aging.

Don'ts:

- Don't rely solely on juices for your nutrition. Juices can be a great supplement to a healthy diet, but they should not be the only source of nutrition.
- Don't use too much fruit in your juices, as it can lead to excess sugar consumption.
- Don't neglect to properly clean and maintain your juicer, as a dirty juicer can harbor harmful bacteria that can impact your health.

Warnings and Advice:

- If you have any underlying health conditions or are taking medication, consult with your healthcare provider before making significant changes to your diet, including adding juices to your routine.
- Be mindful of portion sizes and calorie intake. Juices can be high in calories and sugar, so it's important to consume them in moderation.
- If you experience any adverse effects from juicing, such as bloating, diarrhea, or stomach cramps, reduce your intake or stop juicing altogether and consult with your healthcare provider.

Foods for your Youthful Nutrition Juice

- **Blueberries:** Blueberries are high in antioxidants and can help reduce inflammation, inflammation is linked to aging.

- **Pomegranate:** Pomegranate juice is high in antioxidants and can improve circulation, improved circulation can help keep skin looking youthful.

- **Kale:** Kale is high in antioxidants, vitamin C, and beta-carotene, which can help protect the skin from damage caused by free radicals.

- **Spinach:** Spinach is high in vitamin C, vitamin C is important for collagen production, and can help reduce inflammation.

- **Carrots:** Carrots are high in beta-carotene; beta-carotene is converted to vitamin A in the body and can help prevent wrinkles and improve skin health.

- **Tomatoes:** Tomatoes are high in lycopene; lycopene can help protect the skin from damage caused by the sun.

- **Oranges:** Oranges are high in vitamin C; vitamin C is important for collagen production and can help reduce inflammation.

- **Strawberries:** Strawberries are high in antioxidants; antioxidants can help protect the skin from damage caused by free radicals.

- **Pineapple:** Pineapple is high in vitamin C and bromelain, vitamin C and bromelain can help reduce inflammation and improve digestion.

- **Beetroot:** Beetroot is high in antioxidants and can help improve circulation, which can help keep skin looking youthful.

Boost your Youthful Nutrition Juice

- **Collagen powder:** Collagen is a protein that helps to maintain skin elasticity, improve joint health, and support muscle growth.
- **Chlorella powder:** Chlorella is a type of algae that is high in antioxidants, vitamins, and minerals. Chlorella can help to detoxify the body, boost the immune system, and improve skin health.
- **Maca powder:** Maca is a root vegetable that is high in antioxidants, vitamins, and minerals. Maca can help to improve energy levels, balance hormones, and enhance mood.
- **Ashwagandha powder:** Ashwagandha is an adaptogenic herb that can help to reduce stress, improve cognitive function, and boost the immune system.
- **Turmeric powder:** Turmeric is a spice that is high in antioxidants and has anti-inflammatory properties. Turmeric can help to reduce inflammation, improve brain function, and support healthy digestion.
- **Cinnamon powder:** Cinnamon is a spice that is high in antioxidants and has anti-inflammatory properties. Cinnamon can help to regulate blood sugar levels, reduce inflammation, and improve brain function.
- **Spirulina powder:** Spirulina is a type of blue-green algae that is high in antioxidants, vitamins, and minerals. Spirulina can help to detoxify the body, boost the immune system, and improve energy levels.
- **Matcha powder:** Matcha is a type of green tea that is high in antioxidants and has anti-inflammatory properties. Matcha can help to improve brain function, boost metabolism, and enhance mood.
- **Baobab powder:** Baobab is a fruit that is high in antioxidants, vitamin C, and fiber. Baobab can help to support immune function, improve digestion, and reduce inflammation.
- **Acai powder:** Acai is a berry that is high in antioxidants, vitamins, and minerals. Acai can help to improve skin health, boost the immune system, and reduce inflammation.

Remember to always consult with a healthcare professional before adding any new supplements to your diet.

Purple Juice

Ingredients:

2 cups purple grapes
1/2 cup blueberries
1/2 cup blackberries
1/2 lemon, peeled
1-inch piece of ginger

Instructions:

Wash all the ingredients thoroughly.
Put the ingredients into the juicer and extract the juice.
Pour the juice into a glass and enjoy!

Benefits:

Purple grapes contain resveratrol, a compound that has been linked to anti-aging and longevity.
Blueberries and blackberries are high in antioxidants, which can help prevent cellular damage and slow down the aging process.
Lemon is a good source of vitamin C and can help boost collagen production for healthier skin.
Ginger has anti-inflammatory properties and can help improve skin elasticity.

Nutritional Information:

Calories: 160
Carbohydrates: 41g
Protein: 2g
Fat: 1g
Sugar: 32g
Sodium: 8mg

Pomegranate Juice

Ingredients:

1 pomegranate
1/2 lemon, peeled
1-inch piece of ginger

Instructions:

Wash all the ingredients thoroughly.
Chop the pomegranate into quarters and remove the arils.
Put the ingredients into the juicer and extract the juice.
Pour the juice into a glass and enjoy!

Benefits:

Pomegranate is high in antioxidants, which can help prevent cellular damage and aging.
Lemons are a rich source of vitamin C, known for its ability to promote healthy skin.
Ginger has powerful anti-inflammatory properties that can help reduce pain and inflammation, as well as improve blood circulation.

Nutritional Information:

Calories: 135
Carbohydrates: 32g
Protein: 2g
Fat: 1g
Sugar: 22g
Sodium: 4mg

Pomegranate and Carrot Juice

Ingredients:

1/2 cup pomegranate seeds
3 medium carrots, peeled and chopped
1/2 cucumber
1/2 lemon, peeled

Instructions:

Wash all the ingredients thoroughly.
Chop the carrots and cucumber into small pieces.
Put the ingredients into the juicer and extract the juice.
Pour the juice into a glass and enjoy!

Benefits:

Pomegranate is rich in antioxidants, which can help reduce inflammation
and improve skin health.
Carrots are high in beta-carotene, which can help improve skin elasticity
and reduce the appearance of wrinkles.
Cucumber is high in water and can help hydrate the body and improve skin
texture.
Lemon is a good source of vitamin C, which can help improve collagen
production and reduce the risk of skin damage.

Nutritional Information:

Calories: 118
Carbohydrates: 28g
Protein: 3g
Fat: 1g
Sugar: 16g
Sodium: 77mg

Carrot and Orange Juice

Ingredients:

4 medium carrots, peeled and chopped
2 oranges, peeled and seeded
1-inch piece of fresh ginger, peeled

Instructions:

Wash all the ingredients thoroughly.
Chop the carrots and oranges into small pieces.
Put the ingredients into the juicer and extract the juice.
Pour the juice into a glass and enjoy!

Benefits:

Carrots are rich in antioxidants and can help reduce the signs of aging.
Oranges are high in vitamin C and can help improve skin health.
Ginger has anti-inflammatory properties and can help reduce inflammation
in the body.

Nutritional Information:

Calories: 176
Carbohydrates: 44g
Protein: 4g
Fat: 1g
Sugar: 29g
Sodium: 98mg

Pineapple and Ginger Juice

Ingredients:

2 cups fresh pineapple, chopped
1-inch piece of fresh ginger, peeled

Instructions:

Wash all the ingredients thoroughly.
Chop the pineapple into small pieces.
Put the ingredients into the juicer and extract the juice.
Pour the juice into a glass and enjoy!

Benefits:

Pineapple is high in antioxidants and can help reduce the signs of aging.
Ginger has anti-inflammatory properties and can help improve skin health.

Nutritional Information:

Calories: 200
Carbohydrates: 50g
Protein: 2g
Fat: 1g
Sugar: 38g
Sodium: 2mg

Kale-Cucumber-Pineapple Juice

Ingredients:

1 small bunch of kale, stems removed
1/2 cucumber, peeled and chopped
1/2 pineapple, peeled and chopped
1 inch ginger root, peeled

Instructions:

Wash all the ingredients thoroughly.
Cut the kale into small pieces.
Peel the cucumber and pineapple.
Put the ingredients into the juicer and extract the juice.
Pour the juice into a glass and enjoy!

Benefits:

Kale is high in antioxidants, vitamins A and C, and minerals that support detoxification.
Cucumber contains antioxidants and has diuretic properties that can help to flush toxins out of the body.
Pineapple is high in vitamin C, bromelain, and antioxidants that may help to reduce inflammation and protect against cell damage.
Ginger has anti-inflammatory properties that can help to reduce inflammation in the body.

Nutritional Information:

Calories: 170
Protein: 3g
Fat: 1g
Carbohydrates: 43g
Sugar: 27g
Sodium: 33mg

In conclusion, aging is a complex process that involves a variety of factors, including genetics, lifestyle, and environmental factors. While aging is a natural process that cannot be completely prevented, there are several lifestyle habits that can help slow down the aging process and promote overall health and wellbeing.

Eating a healthy diet that is rich in fruits and vegetables, whole grains, and lean proteins, exercising regularly, managing stress, getting enough sleep, avoiding harmful habits, using sunscreen, and taking steps to reduce exposure to environmental toxins are all effective ways to slow down the aging process.

Juicing can also be a beneficial way to slow down the aging process, as it provides a concentrated source of antioxidants and other nutrients that can help reduce oxidative stress and inflammation in the body. However, it's important to remember that juices should not be relied upon as the sole source of nutrition and should be consumed in moderation.

Incorporating a variety of colorful fruits and vegetables in your juices, considering adding anti-aging superfoods, choosing organic produce, hydrating with plenty of water, and incorporating low-sugar green juices are all effective ways to boost the anti-aging properties of your juices. It's important to be mindful of portion sizes and calorie intake, as juices can be high in calories and sugar.

In addition, it's important to consult with your healthcare provider before making significant changes to your diet, especially if you have underlying health conditions or are taking medication. It's also important to be mindful of any adverse effects from juicing and to reduce your intake or stop juicing altogether if you experience bloating, diarrhea, or stomach cramps.

Overall, by incorporating healthy lifestyle habits and incorporating antioxidant-rich foods into your diet, you can slow down the aging process and promote overall health and wellbeing.

Note: These recipes are not intended to treat or cure any medical condition. Please consult with your healthcare provider before making any significant changes to your diet.

Notes:

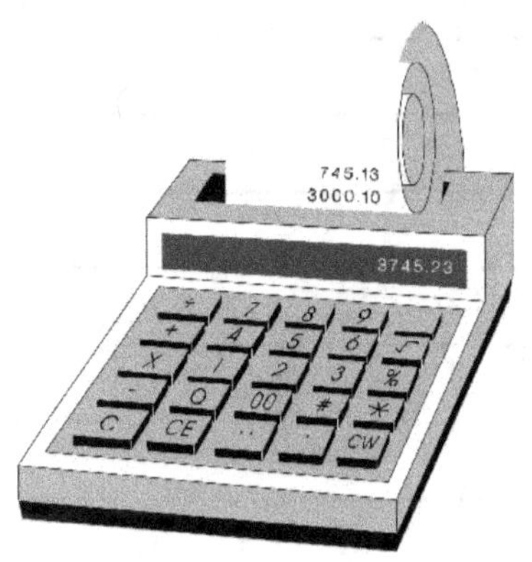

Juicing on a budget

"You are what you eat, so don't be fast, cheap, easy or fake." - Unknown

Is Juicing Expensive?

There are several misconceptions surrounding juicing and its perceived expense. Here are a few:

- **Juicing requires expensive equipment:** While it's true that juicers can be expensive, there are many affordable options on the market. Additionally, you don't necessarily need a juicer to make juice - a blender can also work.

- **Juicing requires expensive ingredients:** While some fruits and vegetables can be costly, there are plenty of affordable options that are great for juicing. In fact, some of the most nutritious fruits and vegetables are also some of the most affordable, such as carrots, apples, and oranges.

- **Juicing is wasteful:** Some people believe that juicing creates a lot of waste, as the pulp and fiber are discarded. However, there are ways to repurpose the pulp, such as adding it to soups or baked goods.

- **Juicing is a fad:** Some people view juicing as a trendy, short-term diet fad. However, incorporating fresh juice into your diet can be a sustainable way to increase your intake of vitamins and minerals, and can be a healthy habit for the long term.

Why juice on a budget?

Juicing is important for many reasons, even if you are on a budget. Here are a few reasons why:

- **Nutrient absorption:** Juicing allows you to consume a large amount of nutrients from fruits and vegetables in an easily digestible form. This helps your body absorb the nutrients more efficiently, leading to better overall health.

- **Hydration:** Juicing can be an excellent way to stay hydrated, especially during hot summer months. Juicing fruits and vegetables can provide a refreshing and hydrating drink that also contains important vitamins and minerals.

- **Variety:** Juicing allows you to consume a wider variety of fruits and vegetables than you might normally eat. This can help you meet your daily recommended intake of essential nutrients.

- **Detoxification:** Some people use juicing to help cleanse their bodies of toxins. While there is limited scientific evidence to support this, many people report feeling better after doing a juice cleanse.

- **Cost savings:** Juicing can be a cost-effective way to consume fruits and vegetables, especially if you shop for produce that is in season or on sale. By juicing at home, you can also save money compared to buying pre-made juices or smoothies from a store.

Overall, juicing is a convenient and efficient way to incorporate more fruits and vegetables into your diet, regardless of your budget.

Foods for you Budget Juice

These fruits and vegetables are often readily available and affordable, making them great options for juicing on a budget.

- **Carrots** - Carrots are rich in antioxidants, vitamins A and C, and beta-carotene, all of which can help to improve vision, skin health, and immunity.
- **Apples** - Apples are a great source of vitamin C and fiber, vitamin C and fiber can help to regulate digestion and lower cholesterol levels.
- **Oranges** - Oranges are packed with vitamin C and flavonoids, vitamin C and flavonoids can help to lower blood pressure and improve heart health.
- **Lemons** - Lemons are a good source of vitamin C and can help to improve skin health and digestion.
- **Cucumbers** - Cucumbers are rich in water and fiber, water and fiber can help to promote hydration and digestion. They also contain vitamin K, which can help to strengthen bones.
- **Celery** - Celery is low in calories and high in fiber, which can help to improve digestion and lower cholesterol levels.
- **Kale** - Kale is a nutrient-dense vegetable that is high in vitamins A, C, and K, and antioxidants. Kale can help to reduce inflammation and improve heart health.
- **Spinach** - Spinach is another nutrient-dense vegetable that is high in vitamins A and C, and antioxidants. Spinach can help to lower blood pressure and improve bone health.
- **Beets** - Beets are rich in nitrates, which can help to improve blood flow and lower blood pressure. Beets also contain antioxidants that can help to reduce inflammation.
- **Sweet Potatoes** - Sweet potatoes are a good source of vitamin A, fiber, and potassium. Vitamin A, fiber, and potassium can help to improve digestion and lower blood pressure.

Boost your Budget Juice

- **Cinnamon:** Cinnamon is a spice that adds a warm, sweet flavor to your juice. It is also known for its anti-inflammatory and antioxidant properties.
- **Ginger:** Ginger has a spicy, zesty flavor that can add a kick to your juice. It is also known for its anti-inflammatory properties and can aid in digestion.
- **Turmeric:** Turmeric is a spice that has a warm, slightly bitter taste. It is also known for its anti-inflammatory and antioxidant properties.
- **Chia seeds:** Chia seeds are small, inexpensive seeds that can be added to your juice for extra fiber and protein. They also contain omega-3 fatty acids, which are good for heart health.
- **Flaxseed:** Flaxseed is another inexpensive seed that can be added to your juice for extra fiber and protein. It also contains omega-3 fatty acids.
- **Lemon juice:** Lemon juice can be added to your juice for a tangy flavor. It is also high in vitamin C and antioxidants.
- **Apple cider vinegar:** Apple cider vinegar can add a tangy flavor to your juice and is also known for its potential health benefits, such as aiding in digestion and regulating blood sugar levels.
- **Cayenne pepper:** Cayenne pepper can add a spicy kick to your juice and is also known for its potential to boost metabolism and aid in digestion.
- **Beet greens:** Beet greens are the leafy tops of beets and can be added to your juice for extra nutrients, such as vitamin C and potassium.
- **Parsley:** Parsley is an herb that can be added to your juice for a fresh, slightly bitter flavor. It is also high in vitamin K and antioxidants.

It is important to note that while these additives can be inexpensive, some of them may not be readily available in all regions or may be seasonal. Additionally, it is recommended to consult with a healthcare professional before adding any new supplements or ingredients to your diet.

Carrot-Apple-Beet Juice

Ingredients:

2 medium-sized carrots
1 small apple
1 small beet

Instructions:

Wash and prepare the ingredients.
Cut them into small pieces that can easily fit into your juicer.
Put the ingredients into the juicer and extract the juice.
Pour the juice into a glass and enjoy!

Benefits:

Carrots are high in antioxidants and vitamin A, which promote healthy vision and skin.
Apples are rich in fiber and vitamin C that can support digestive health and immune function.
Beets contain nitrates that can help improve blood flow and lower blood pressure.

Nutrition:

Calories: 135
Carbohydrates: 33g
Protein: 2g
Fat: 0g

Pineapple-Cucumber-Lime Juice

Ingredients:

1/2 small pineapple
1/2 cucumber
1 lime

Instructions:

Wash and prepare the ingredients.
Cut the pineapple and cucumber into small pieces that can easily fit into
your juicer.
Put the ingredients into the juicer and extract the juice.
Pour the juice into a glass and enjoy!

Benefits:

Pineapples contain bromelain, an enzyme that aids digestion and reduces
inflammation.
Cucumbers are hydrating and rich in vitamins and minerals, including
vitamin K and potassium.
Limes are high in vitamin C and antioxidants, which support immune
function and skin health.

Nutrition:

Calories: 116
Carbohydrates: 30g
Protein: 2g
Fat: 0g

Spinach-Apple-Lemon Juice

Ingredients:

2 cups spinach
2 small apples
1/2 lemon

Instructions:

Wash and prepare the ingredients.
Cut the apples into small pieces that can easily fit into your juicer.
Put the ingredients into the juicer and extract the juice.
Pour the juice into a glass and enjoy!

Benefits:

Spinach is a good source of iron and other essential minerals, as well as antioxidants that protect against cell damage.
Apples are high in fiber and vitamin C, which support digestive health and immune function.
Lemons are alkalizing and contain compounds that can help reduce inflammation.

Nutrition:

Calories: 140
Carbohydrates: 35g
Protein: 3g
Fat: 0g

Beet-Orange-Ginger Juice

Ingredients:

1 medium-sized beet
2 oranges
1/2-inch fresh ginger

Instructions:

Wash and prepare the ingredients.
Cut the beet and oranges into small pieces that can easily fit into your juicer.
Peel and grate the ginger.
Put the ingredients into the juicer and extract the juice.
Pour the juice into a glass and enjoy!

Benefits:

Beets are high in nitrates that can help improve blood flow and lower blood pressure.
Oranges are rich in vitamin C and other antioxidants, which support immune function and skin health.
Ginger has anti-inflammatory properties and can help soothe digestion.

Nutrition:

Calories: 201
Carbohydrates: 49g
Protein: 4g
Fat: 1

Notes:

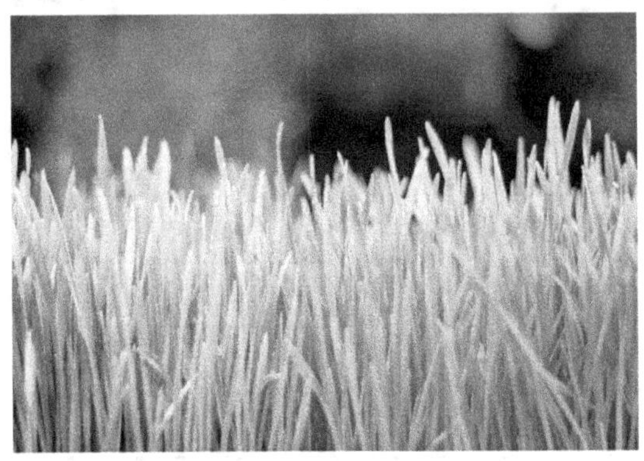

Nourish Your Body

Some of our favorite juices

"Juicing is a powerful tool for detoxifying your body, boosting your energy levels, and improving your overall health and well-being." - Unknown

Vegetable Cleanse Juice

Ingredients:

4 medium tomatoes
4 large carrots
1 red bell pepper
2 stalks celery
1 small beet, peeled
1/2 lemon, peeled
1-inch piece of fresh ginger, peeled

Instructions:

Wash all the ingredients thoroughly.
Chop the tomatoes, carrots, bell pepper, and celery into small pieces.
Put the ingredients into the juicer and extract the juice.
Pour the juice into a glass and enjoy!

Benefits:

Tomatoes contain high levels of lycopene, a potent antioxidant that has been linked to a reduced risk of cancer and heart disease.
Carrots are high in vitamin A, which can help improve vision and skin health.
Red bell peppers are high in vitamin C, which can help boost the immune system and promote healthy skin.
Celery is high in antioxidants and can help lower inflammation in the body.
Beets are an excellent source of nitrates, which the body converts into nitric oxide. This has been shown to increase blood flow and reduce blood pressure, making beets a beneficial part of any diet.
Lemon is high in vitamin C and can help improve digestion.
Ginger has powerful anti-inflammatory properties that can help reduce pain and inflammation, as well as improve blood circulation.

Nutritional Information:

Calories: 174
Carbohydrates: 41g
Protein: 6g
Fat: 1g
Sugar: 22g
Sodium: 326mg

Veggie Vitality Juice

Ingredients:

1 large cucumber
2 stalks celery
2 large carrots
1 small beet, peeled
1 small green apple, cored
1/2 lemon, peeled
1/2-inch piece of fresh ginger, peeled
Handful of spinach leaves
Handful of kale leaves

Instructions:

Wash all the ingredients thoroughly.
Chop the cucumber, celery, carrots, beet, and apple into small pieces.
Put the ingredients into the juicer and extract the juice.
Pour the juice into a glass and enjoy!

Benefits:

Cucumber is hydrating and can help reduce inflammation in the body.
Celery is high in antioxidants and can help lower inflammation in the body.
Carrots are high in vitamin A, which can help improve vision and skin health.
Beets are an excellent source of nitrates, which the body converts into nitric oxide.
This has been shown to increase blood flow and reduce blood pressure, making
beets a beneficial part of any diet.
Green apple is high in fiber and can help improve digestion.
Lemon is high in vitamin C and can help improve digestion.
Ginger has powerful anti-inflammatory properties that can help reduce pain and
inflammation, as well as improve blood circulation.
Spinach and kale are high in antioxidants, vitamins, and minerals that can help
support overall health and well-being.

Nutritional Information:
Calories: 147
Carbohydrates: 36g
Protein: 5g
Fat: 1g
Sugar: 21g
Sodium: 221mg

Rooted in Health Juice

Ingredients:

2 large carrots
2 stalks celery
1 small beet, peeled
1 small green apple, cored
1/2 lemon, peeled
1/2-inch piece of fresh ginger, peeled
1 cup baby spinach

Instructions:

Wash all the ingredients thoroughly.
Chop the carrots, celery, beet, and apple into small pieces.
Put the ingredients into the juicer and extract the juice.
Pour the juice into a glass and enjoy!

Benefits:

Carrots are high in vitamin A, which can help improve vision and skin health.
Celery is high in antioxidants and can help lower inflammation in the body.
Beets are an excellent source of nitrates, which the body converts into nitric oxide.
This has been shown to increase blood flow and reduce blood pressure, making
beets a beneficial part of any diet.
Green apple is high in fiber and can help improve digestion.
Lemon is high in vitamin C and can help improve digestion.
Ginger has powerful anti-inflammatory properties that can help reduce pain and
inflammation, as well as improve blood circulation.
Spinach is high in iron and can help support healthy blood cells.

Nutritional Information:

Calories: 103
Carbohydrates: 26g
Protein: 3g
Fat: 1g
Sugar: 16g
Sodium: 180m

Green Refresh Juice

Ingredients:

1/2 cucumber
1 Granny Smith apple
3 stalks of celery

Instructions:

Wash all ingredients thoroughly.
Cut the cucumber and apple into small pieces that will fit into your juicer.
Cut the celery stalks into smaller pieces as well.
Put the ingredients into the juicer and extract the juice.
Pour the juice into a glass and enjoy!

Benefits:

Cucumbers are high in antioxidants, can help reduce inflammation and hydrate the body.
Granny Smith apples are rich in vitamins and minerals, can help boost the immune system and improve digestion.
Celery contains anti-inflammatory properties, that can help lower blood pressure, and improve overall heart health.

Nutritional Information:

Calories: 70
Carbohydrates: 18g
Protein: 1g
Fat: 0.5g

Island Delight

Ingredients:

1/4 pineapple, peeled and chopped
1/4 papaya, peeled and chopped

Instructions:

Wash the fruits thoroughly.
Peel and chop the pineapple and papaya into small pieces.
Put the ingredients into the juicer and extract the juice.
Pour the juice into a glass and enjoy!

Benefits:

Pineapple is rich in vitamin C, which is important for a healthy immune system and may help protect against cancer.
Papaya contains an enzyme called papain that can help improve digestion and reduce inflammation.

Nutrition information:

Calories: 120
Carbohydrates: 31g
Protein: 2g
Fat: 1g

Beet-Apple-Orange Juice

Ingredients:

1 large beet
1 apple, cored and chopped
1 orange, peeled and chopped

Instructions:

Wash and prep the beet, apple, and orange.
Cut the beet and apple into small pieces that fit into your juicer.
Peel the orange and remove any seeds.
Put the ingredients into the juicer and extract the juice.
Pour the juice into a glass and enjoy!

Benefits:

Beets are rich in nitrates, which can help lower blood pressure and improve blood flow. They also contain betaine, which can help reduce inflammation and protect against liver damage.
Apples are a good source of fiber and vitamin C. They also contain polyphenols, which have been shown to have antioxidant and anti-inflammatory effects.
Oranges are rich in vitamin C, which can help improve skin health and boost the immune system. They also contain flavonoids, which can help improve heart health and lower the risk of chronic diseases.

Nutritional:

Calories: 170
Carbohydrates: 43g
Protein: 3g
Fat: 1g

Tips to stay healthy while juicing

In addition to the general healthy lifestyle habits I have mentioned, here are some tips specifically for promoting healthy aging through juicing:

1. Incorporate a variety of fruits and vegetables into your juices. Aim for a colorful mix of produce to ensure you are getting a variety of nutrients.

2. Choose fruits and vegetables that are high in antioxidants, such as berries, leafy greens, and beets.

3. Add in herbs and spices, such as ginger, turmeric, and cinnamon, which have anti-inflammatory properties and can help reduce oxidative stress.

4. Use a slow juicer to minimize heat and oxidation, which can damage nutrients.

5. Drink your juice immediately or store it in an airtight container in the refrigerator for no more than 24 hours to maximize nutrient content.

6. Consider doing a juice cleanse or incorporating a juice fast into your routine to help eliminate toxins from the body.

7. Stay hydrated by drinking plenty of water in addition to your juices.

8. Maintain a balanced diet that includes whole foods and lean proteins in addition to your juices.

9. Get regular exercise to maintain muscle mass and mobility.

10. Get regular check-ups with your healthcare provider to monitor any age-related health issues and address them promptly.

Notes:

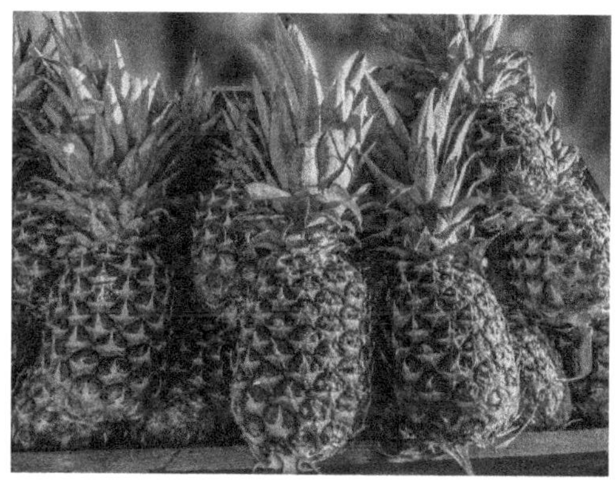

Create a juicing routine that works for your lifestyle

"Juicing is not just a fad, it's a way of life. It's a way to stay healthy, happy, and full of energy." - Unknown

Make it work for you

Creating a juicing routine that works for your lifestyle can help you maintain healthy habits and reap the benefits of juicing. Here are some tips for creating a juicing routine that works for you:

- **Start small:** If you're new to juicing, start with one juice a day and gradually increase the frequency as you get used to it.

- **Plan ahead:** Decide which days of the week you'll juice, what time of day you'll juice, and what ingredients you'll need.

- **Prep ahead:** Wash and chop your fruits and vegetables ahead of time so that they're ready to go when you're ready to juice.

- **Experiment:** Try different combinations of fruits and vegetables to find what you like and what works for your body.

- **Be consistent:** Stick to your juicing routine even when life gets busy or stressful.

- **Listen to your body:** Pay attention to how your body feels after you juice and adjust your routine accordingly.

- **Stay motivated:** Set goals for yourself, such as a certain number of juices per week, and reward yourself when you meet those goals.

- **Make it enjoyable:** Play music, listen to a podcast, or involve friends or family to make juicing a fun and social activity.

Remember, the most important thing is to create a routine that works for you and fits into your lifestyle. With time and practice, you'll find what works best for your body and enjoy the many benefits of juicing.

Waste?

Juicing is a great way to get more fruits and vegetables into your diet, but it can also generate a lot of waste in the form of pulp. Here are some creative ways to use juice pulp and minimize waste:

- **Make veggie burgers:** Use pulp from carrots, beets, and other root vegetables to make veggie burgers. Mix the pulp with cooked grains like quinoa, breadcrumbs, and seasonings. Then form into patties and bake or fry.

- **Make crackers:** Spread out the pulp on a baking sheet, sprinkle with herbs and spices, and bake at a low temperature until crispy.

- **Make vegetable broth:** Boil the pulp with water and seasonings to make a nutrient-rich vegetable broth.

- **Add to soups and stews:** Use the pulp in place of, or in addition to, vegetables in your favorite soup or stew recipes.

- **Add to smoothies:** Add a spoonful of pulp to your smoothies for added fiber and nutrition.

- **Use as a thickener:** Use fruit pulp to thicken sauces, jams, and other recipes that call for fruit.

- **Feed it to your pets:** Many pets enjoy vegetable pulp as a healthy snack.

- **Compost it:** If all else fails, compost the pulp to enrich your garden soil.

By using juice pulp in creative ways, you can reduce waste and make the most of your fruits and vegetables.

Time saving ideas

Juicing can be a time-consuming process, but there are several hacks and time-saving tips that can make it easier and more efficient. Here are some of them:

1. **Prep ahead:** Wash and chop your fruits and vegetables ahead of time so that they are ready to go when you're ready to juice.

2. **Juice in batches:** Make a large batch of juice at once and store it in the refrigerator or freezer for later use.

3. **Use a high-speed juicer:** High-speed juicers can process fruits and vegetables faster than other types of juicers.

4. **Clean as you go:** Clean your juicer immediately after use to avoid a buildup of pulp and to make the cleaning process quicker and easier.

5. **Use a strainer or nut milk bag:** Using a strainer or nut milk bag to strain the juice can make the process quicker and eliminate the need to clean the juicer as frequently.

6. **Mix and match:** Try mixing and matching different fruits and vegetables to create new flavors and to increase the variety of nutrients in your juice.

7. **Freeze fruits and vegetables:** Freeze fruits and vegetables that are about to spoil, and use them in your next batch of juice.

8. **Experiment with recipes:** Experiment with different recipes to find what works best for you and your taste preferences.

By implementing these hacks and time-saving tips, you can make juicing a more efficient and enjoyable process.

Notes:

Notes:

Notes:

Suggested Reading List

1. **"Medical Medium"** by Anthony William
2. **"The Plant Paradox"** by Steven R. Gundry
3. **"How Not to Die"** by Michael Greger
4. **"The Whole30"** by Melissa Hartwig Urban and Dallas Hartwig
5. **"Clean Gut"** by Alejandro Junger
6. **"The Paleo Solution"** by Robb Wolf
7. **"Eat to Live"** by Joel Fuhrman
8. **"The Wahls Protocol"** by Terry Wahls
9. **"The 4-Hour Body"** by Tim Ferriss
10. **"The Bulletproof Diet"** by Dave Asprey
11. **"The Hormone Reset Diet"** by Sara Gottfried
12. **"The Blood Sugar Solution"** by Mark Hyman
13. **"The UltraMind Solution"** by Mark Hyman
14. **"The End of Diabetes"** by Joel Fuhrman
15. **"The Longevity Diet"** by Valter Longo
16. **"The Juicing Bible"** by Pat Crocker
17. **"The Big Book of Juices"** by Natalie Savona
18. **"Juicing for Life: A Guide to the Benefits of Fresh Fruit and Vegetable Juicing"** by Cherie Calbom and Maureen Keane
19. **"The Complete Idiot's Guide to Juicing"** by Ellen Brown
20. **"Superfood Juices & Smoothies: 100 Delicious and Mega-Nutritious Recipes from the World's Most Powerful Superfoods"** by Julie Morris
21. **"Juice Fasting and Detoxification: Use the Healing Power of Fresh Juice to Feel Young and Look Great"** by Steve Meyerowitz
22. **"The Everything Juicing Book: All You Need to Create Delicious Juices for Your Optimum Health"** by Carole Jacobs and Patrice Johnson
23. **"Juice It!: Energizing Blends for Today's Juicers"** by Robin Asbell
24. **"The Juicing Detox Diet"** by Christine Bailey
25. **"The Juicing Diet: Drink Your Way to Weight Loss, Cleansing, Health, and Beauty"** by Sonoma Press

Conclusion

Juicing can be an incredibly beneficial way to nourish your body and boost your energy. Whether you are looking to improve your heart health, circulation, reverse diabetes, or aging, or simply cleanse your system, there are a variety of recipes and ingredients that can help you achieve your goals.

Feel free to conduct your own experiments and try out new combinations! Juicing is a fun and creative way to incorporate a variety of fruits and vegetables into your diet, and there is no one "right" way to do it. Try out different combinations, experiment with new ingredients, and see what works best for you and your body.

Keep in mind that while juicing can be beneficial, it's important to consider it as a supplement to a well-rounded healthy lifestyle. It is important to also incorporate regular exercise, plenty of rest, and a balanced diet to achieve optimal health and wellbeing. With dedication and a willingness to explore, you can use juicing as a tool to help you achieve your health and wellness goals. So go ahead and have fun with juicing - your body will thank you for it!

Note: These recipes are not intended to treat or cure any medical condition. Please consult with your healthcare provider before making any significant changes to your diet.

Sources:

- Healthline. (n.d.). 20 Best Fruits to Eat for Breakfast. https://www.healthline.com/nutrition/best-fruits-for-breakfast
- Medical News Today. (2021). 10 healthful fruits to eat during pregnancy. https://www.medicalnewstoday.com/articles/324458#Fruit-to-eat-during-pregnancy
- "Juicing: What are the Health Benefits?" Mayo Clinic, 2021. https://www.mayoclinic.org/healthy-lifestyle/nutrition-and-healthy-eating/in-depth/juicing/art-20047964
- "Juicing: Benefits, Risks, and Recipes," WebMD, 2020. https://www.webmd.com/diet/features/juicing-health-risks-and-benefits
- "The Pros and Cons of Juicing," Harvard Health Publishing, 2019. https://www.health.harvard.edu/staying-healthy/the-pros-and-cons-of-juicing
- "10 Time-Saving Tips for Juicing," Healthline, https://www.healthline.com/nutrition/time-saving-tips-for-juicing
- "5 Time-Saving Tips for Juicing," Reboot with Joe, https://www.rebootwithjoe.com/5-time-saving-tips-for-juicing/
- "What to Do With Leftover Juice Pulp," Healthline, https://www.healthline.com/nutrition/what-to-do-with-juice-pulp
- "5 Ways to Use Leftover Juice Pulp," The Spruce Eats, https://www.thespruceeats.com/leftover-juice-pulp-uses-3376483
- "Juice Pulp Recipes: 20 Delicious Uses for Leftover Juice Pulp," Green Press, https://greenpress.co/blogs/news/20-ways-to-use-leftover-juice-pulp
- Healthline - https://www.healthline.com/nutrition/detox-juice-recipes)
- Eatingwell - https://www.eatingwell.com/
- Food Network - https://www.foodnetwork.com/recipes/food-network-kitchen/

- Harvard Health Publishing. (2018). The truth about juicing. https://www.health.harvard.edu/staying-healthy/the-truth-about-juicing
- Medical News Today. (2021). What are the benefits of juicing? https://www.medicalnewstoday.com/articles/323828
- Healthline. (2021). Juicing: What are the benefits? https://www.healthline.com/nutrition/juicing-benefits
- Bunner, A. E., Wells, C. L., Gonzales, J., & Agarwal, U. (2014). A dietary intervention for chronic diabetic neuropathy pain: a randomized controlled pilot study. Nutrition & diabetes, 4(4), e132.
- https://doi.org/10.1038/nutd.2014.28
- Shehata, A. M., & Schrader, L. F. (2018). Juicing for Health: A Review of the Benefits of a Juicing Lifestyle. Current opinion in food science, 22, 89–94. https://doi.org/10.1016/j.cofs.2018.04.001
- Thompson, L. (2014). Nutrition therapy recommendations for the management of adults with diabetes. Diabetes Spectrum, 27(4), 277-284. https://doi.org/10.2337/diaspect.27.4.277
- "10 Foods That Are Good for Your Heart," Healthline, https://www.healthline.com/nutrition/heart-healthy-foods#TOC_TITLE_HDR_2
- "5 Heart-Healthy Juices to Lower High Blood Pressure," Step to Health, https://steptohealth.com/5-heart-healthy-juices-to-lower-high-blood-pressure/
- Blue Zones - Lessons From the World's Longest Lived https://www.ncbi.nlm.nih.gov/pmc/articles/PMC6125071/
- Influence of refractive error on pupillary dynamics in the normal and mild traumatic brain injury (mTBI) populations https://www.ncbi.nlm.nih.gov/pmc/articles/PMC5904777/
- A tandem simulation framework for predicting mapping quality https://www.ncbi.nlm.nih.gov/pmc/articles/PMC5557537/
- Epithelial insulin receptor expression–prognostic relevance in colorectal cancer https://www.ncbi.nlm.nih.gov/pmc/articles/PMC6331016/
- Pharmacotherapy for acute mania and disconcordance with treatment guidelines: bipolar mania pathway survey (BIPAS) in mainland China https://www.ncbi.nlm.nih.gov/pmc/articles/PMC4061451/
- Oligomeric Status and Nucleotide Binding Properties of the Plastid ATP/ADP Transporter 1: Toward a Molecular Understanding of the Transport Mechanism https://www.ncbi.nlm.nih.gov/pmc/articles/PMC3306366/

- Healthline. (2021). 7 Tips for Making Healthy Juicing a Habit. Retrieved from https://www.healthline.com/nutrition/healthy-juicing-tips
- WebMD. (2021). Juicing: How Healthy Is It? Retrieved from https://www.webmd.com/diet/features/juicing-health-risks-and-benefits
- Food Network. (n.d.). Juicing: How to Get Started. Retrieved from https://www.foodnetwork.com/healthyeats/healthy-tips/2013/04/juicing-how-to-get-started
- EatingWell. (2019). The Beginner's Guide to Juicing. Retrieved from https://www.eatingwell.com/article/15872/the-beginners-guide-to-juicing/
- Mayo Clinic. (2020). Water: How much should you drink every day? Retrieved from https://www.mayoclinic.org/healthy-lifestyle/nutrition-and-healthy-eating/in-depth/water/art-20044256
- Harvard Health Publishing. (2019). Juicing: What are the health benefits? Retrieved from https://www.health.harvard.edu/staying-healthy/juicing-what-are-the-health-benefits
- "6 Tips to Make Juicing for Health Safe and Delicious." Harvard Health Publishing, Harvard Medical School, 22 June 2020, https://www.health.harvard.edu/staying-healthy/6-tips-to-make-juicing-for-health-safe-and-delicious
- "The Do's and Don'ts of Juicing While Fasting." Healthline, 27 June 2019, https://www.healthline.com/health/food-nutrition/juicing-while-fasting
- "10 Tips for Juicing on a Budget" by Jessica Chou, Shape Magazine, https://www.shape.com/healthy-eating/cooking-ideas/juicing-budget-tips
- "Juicing on a Budget: Tips and Recipes" by Linda Wagner, The Huffington Post, https://www.huffpost.com/entry/juicing-on-a-budget-tips-_b_8586480
- "Juicer Buying Guide" Consumer Reports - https://www.consumerreports.org/cro/juicers/buying-guide/index.htm
- "How to Choose the Best Juicer for You" by Kelli Foster https://www.thekitchn.com/how-to-choose-the-best-juicer-for-you-244450
- "Fruits and Vegetables to Avoid While Juicing" by Kirsten Nunez, Healthline, June 19, 2020.
- "5 Fruits and Vegetables You Should Not Juice" by Samantha Clayton, Herbalife Nutrition, August 26, 2019.

- American Diabetes Association. (2021). Food and Fitness. https://www.diabetes.org/nutrition
- Harvard Health Publishing. (2021). Diet and Diabetes: A Personalized Approach. https://www.health.harvard.edu/diabetes/diet-and-diabetes-a-personalized-approach
- Mayo Clinic. (2021). Diabetes diet: Create your healthy-eating plan. https://www.mayoclinic.org/diseases-conditions/diabetes/in-depth/diabetes-diet/art-20044295
- American Heart Association. (2021). Healthy Fats. https://www.heart.org/en/healthy-living/healthy-eating/eat-smart/fats/healthy-fats
- American Heart Association. (2021). Know Your Fats. https://www.heart.org/en/healthy-living/healthy-eating/eat-smart/fats/know-your-fats
- Harvard T.H. Chan School of Public Health. (2021). Fruits and Vegetables. https://www.hsph.harvard.edu/nutritionsource/what-should-you-eat/vegetables-and-fruits/
- Harvard T.H. Chan School of Public Health. (2021). Whole Grains. https://www.hsph.harvard.edu/nutritionsource/what-should-you-eat/whole-grains/
- Mayo Clinic. (2021). Heart-healthy diet: 8 steps to prevent heart disease. https://www.mayoclinic.org/diseases-conditions/heart-disease/in-depth/heart-healthy-diet/art-20047702
- Harvard Health Publishing. (2018). Juicing: Healthy detox or diet trap? https://www.health.harvard.edu/staying-healthy/juicing-healthy-detox-or-diet-trap
- Healthline. (2021). The 7 Best Anti-Aging Foods for Your Skin. https://www.healthline.com/nutrition/7-anti-aging-foods
- Medical News Today. (2020). What are the benefits of drinking water? https://www.medicalnewstoday.com/articles/290814
- "Juicing for Health: 10 Do's and Don'ts of Juicing," Healthline, https://www.healthline.com/nutrition/juicing-for-health
- "10 Rules for a Successful Juice Cleanse," EatingWell, https://www.eatingwell.com/article/287287/10-rules-for-a-successful-juice-cleanse/
- "Juicing: What You Need to Know," Mayo Clinic, https://www.mayoclinic.org/healthy-lifestyle/nutrition-and-healthy-eating/in-depth/juicing/art-20047964
- "Foods That Improve Your Circulation," Healthline, https://www.healthline.com/nutrition/foods-that-improve-circulation#TOC_TITLE_HDR_6
- "6 Foods That Improve Circulation," Medical News Today, https://www.medicalnewstoday.com/articles/323335

- "Heart-Healthy Eating: Shopping and Cooking," American Heart Association, https://www.heart.org/en/healthy-living/healthy-eating/eat-smart/nutrition-basics/heart-healthy-eating-shopping-and-cooking
- "Juicing: What are the health benefits?" Mayo Clinic, https://www.mayoclinic.org/healthy-lifestyle/nutrition-and-healthy-eating/in-depth/juicing/art-20047374
- American Diabetes Association. (2022). Top Ten Low-Glycemic Fruits. https://www.diabetes.org/healthy-living/recipes-nutrition/understanding-carbs/top-ten-low-glycemic-fruits
- Gomes, J. M., Costa, J. A., Alfenas, R. de C. G., & de Cássia Gonçalves Alfenas, R. (2017). Metabolic endotoxemia and diabetes mellitus: A systematic review. Metabolism, 68, 133-144. https://doi.org/10.1016/j.metabol.2016.11.006
- Pal, S., & Khossousi, A. (2013). The effect of a low glycemic index breakfast on blood glucose, insulin, and appetite in patients with type 2 diabetes. Journal of the American College of Nutrition, 32(4), 296-300. https://doi.org/10.1080/07315724.2013.816614
- "The History of Juicing: From Ancient Egypt to Modern Times" by Dr. Axe (https://draxe.com/nutrition/the-history-of-juicing/)
- "The Juicing Craze: Is It Really Healthy?" by Time Magazine (https://time.com/3992496/the-juicing-craze-is-it-really-healthy/)